The Clinical Nurse Specialist:
Issues in Practice

The Clinical Nurse Specialist:
Issues in Practice

Edited by

DEBRA HUMPHRIS

MA, RGN, DipN(Londs), RNT

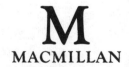

MACMILLAN

First published 1994 by
THE MACMILLAN PRESS LTD
Houndmills, Basingstoke, Hampshire RG21 2XS
and London
Companies and representatives
throughout the world

ISBN 0–333–59466–5

A catalogue record for this book is available
from the British Library

Printed in Great Britain by Mackays of Chatham, PLC. Chatham, Kent

Fiona Cameron
Hospital Manager
Petersfield Hospital

Debra Humphris
Clinical Audit Co-ordinator
South West Thames Regional Health Authority
Formerly Course Leader ENB AO5 Diabetes Nurse Specialist Course

Sheila Mackie Bailey
Freelance Lecturer/Consultant

Sarah Smart
Service Manager
Department of Urology
St Mary's Hospital, Portsmouth

Caroline Soar
Nurse Teacher
Department of Professional Development
West Sussex College of Nursing & Midwifery

Stephen Graham Wright
Director
The European Nursing Development Agency
Tameside General Hospital

EDITOR'S NOTE

The word *nursing* is used, for simplicity, throughout this text, to include nurses, midwives and health visitors.

CONTENTS

Clinical Nurse Specialists are a powerhouse for practice, their energy and drive providing a vital contribution to the quality and development of nursing practice centred on the needs of individuals. Amongst all Clinical Nurse Specialists there are common areas of practice. Therefore the intention of this book is to deal with these commonalities within the context of the United Kingdom health care service, and consequentially shaped around the key roles of the Clinical Nurse Specialist.

Over the last decade, nursing in the United Kingdom has witnessed a major development and expansion in the number of Clinical Nurse Specialists. These posts have been developed across a wide range of practice areas, with practitioners having a variety of levels of preparation, resulting in a very diverse group. This book is aimed at all Clinical Nurse Specialists, no matter what their speciality, and others who aspire to be so. It is hoped that the exploration of the areas of commonality among Clinical Nurse Specialists may encourage the debate which will lead to recognition of the benefits achieved by peer collaboration.

Rarely have so many factors in the wider picture of health care presented one group within nursing with such an opportunity to flourish and demonstrate the tangible worth of its contribution. The commitment to a range of initiatives, aimed at constantly improving the quality of the National Health Service, such as the Health of the Nation, the Patients' Charter and reducing Junior Hospital Doctors' hours, all present Clinical Nurse Specialists with unrivalled opportunities. The *raison d'être* of the role is to provide a high quality individualised service which is effective for the individual service-user. Clinical Nurse Specialists usually provide a service across a wide range of clinical areas within health care organisations, consequently they are both intra and entrepreneurial, working constantly to enhance the quality of the service provided to the population.

A central debate concerning the Clinical Nurse Specialist role is the need to explore the very essence of role *specialism*, and, therefore, to set out the fundamental structure of the role. In the first chapter I have highlighted not only the use of role theory and role definition statements, but also some of the tensions and dilemmas which may face every Clinical Nurse Specialist. One such dilemma is the differentiation between *speciality* and *specialism*, for it could be argued that as soon as nurses qualify and work within a particular area of care that they are in a speciality, and have started to specialise. However, does this make them specialists?

A major role of the Clinical Nurse Specialist is that of direct care, and in the second chapter Fiona Cameron explores some of the models of Specialist Practice. Having worked as a Clinical Nurse Specialist in elderly care, Fiona has dealt at first hand with the complex issues related to the operationalisation of the role. The purpose of the chapter is to explore differing models and frameworks which may be utilised by the Nurse Specialist in organising and operationalising the role. Fundamental to that exploration is some discussion aimed at explicating the differences between theoretical models and conceptual models.

Central to professional nursing practice without question is a research base, and in Chapter 3 Sheila Mackie Bailey examines the role of the Clinical Nurse Specialist in relation to the generation or motivation of the application of research in practice.

An important element of Clinical Nurse Specialist practice is its role as an educator, which is an element that consumes a considerable amount of the role, involving as it does clients, carers and colleagues. In Chapter 4 Caroline Soar and I have not set out to deal with the 'how' to educate, as these issues are dealt with extensively elsewhere in the literature. The intention of the chapter is to explore some of the issues related to the educator role, and in so doing, illustrate some of the dilemmas and contradictions faced by the Clinical Nurse Specialist. One intention is to question a number of assumptions and stimulate debate, as well as asking how effective is educational activity.

The development of the Clinical Nurse Specialist role, both in nature and number brings with it not only issues of professional accountability, but also wider legal and ethical implications. Caroline Soar, as Secretary to the Royal College of Nursing Ethics Forum, has an extensive knowledge of ethical and legal issues in clinical practice. In Chapter 5 she examines these, and the dilemmas such issues raise for Clinical Nurse Specialists.

An issue uppermost in the minds of many Clinical Nurse Specialists is the responsibility upon them to evaluate their role. We all have a professional responsibility to engage in the evaluation of the service we deliver; for Clinical Nurse Specialists it may be to justify the role and its expenditure against a perceived threat of a reduction in services. Equally, evaluation may be about taking the opportunity to develop the role and its place within the Provider Unit, and thus attract extra resources. In Chapter 6 Sarah Smart, formally a Clinical Nurse Specialist, explores a range of strategies that present the Clinical Nurse Specialist with an opportunity to reflect and examine the services currently offered, and identify what is still required.

An increasing number of nurses in the United Kingdom have now adopted the title 'Consultant Nurse' or 'Nurse Consultant'. These two terms are themselves symbolic of the lack of clarity about what constitutes the role. There appears to be little clear consensus as to the role of consultant nurses, what their functions are, what educational background or experience they should have, what pay scales are appropriate, or how they differ from other, but clearly related, roles such as the Clinical Nurse Specialist. In the final chapter Stephen Graham Wright, Director of The European Nursing Development Agency, explores the concept of the Nurse Consultant, whether it is fact or fiction, and the relationship to the Clinical Nurse Specialist's role.

To date, there has been no British text which addresses the common issues of importance to all Clinical Nurse Specialists, regardless of their area of practice. In all the chapters, direct links to practice have been made with the use of examples based on the contributor's own experience.

Our aim is to inform and enhance the debate about the range of issues common to all Clinical Nurse Specialists. The vast majority of texts on Clinical Nurse Specialism are north American in origin, with the associated cross-cultural translation issues this brings. Clearly, the Clinical Nurse Specialist role within the United Kingdom National Health Service is subject to a range of pressures, including the implementation of the NHS & Community Care Act 1990, the Post Registration Education and Practice recommendations, the New Deal on junior Doctors' hours, workforce re-profiling, and the Scope of Professional Practice. All of these present both threats and opportunities to Clinical Nurse Specialists. What we have set out to do is to raise the debate on some of these issues, but we have by no means dealt with them all. We are however all clear about the vital contribution Clinical Nurse Specialists have to make to the continuing development of the quality of individualised patient/client care.

Debra Humphris
1993

CHAPTER ONE

The basis of role specialism in nursing

Debra Humphris

The 20th Century has witnessed the rapid and dramatic expansion of knowledge, with resulting social and technological changes. One consequence of these changes has been the development of specialisation of knowledge and skills. This has resulted in a greater differentiation of the workforce, with.specialisation becoming an almost inevitable occurrence in most professions (Lane, 1985). Indeed, the need for practitioners who possess specialist nursing skills and knowledge has long been recognised, and used in evidence to confirm nursing's professional status (Jolley, 1989; International Council of Nurses, 1992).

WHY SPECIALISTS?

The movement to put the organisation of work in Western industrialised societies on a more specialist base was instigated by Max Weber (Hewa and Hetherington, 1990) – work on the theory of rationalisation. In this, Weber suggested that instrumental rational action, which he defined as "based on purely rational choice among possible means to obtain certain defined goals," would become dominant in modern industrial society. In the National Health Service the evidence of such rationalisation can be seen, as medicine constantly develops new technologies and resulting specialist branches, in its search for the ability to deal with all ill-health and enhancement of good health. The applicability of Weberian theory to the organisation of medical and nursing care was examined by Hewa and Hetherington (1990). They discovered a fundamental paradox in the Weberian approach, namely the tension between a medical–technological approach, which places its emphasis on rational, mechanistic action to solve problems of illness, and the resulting loss of human relations

(Kerrison, 1990). For Hewa and Hetherington (1990) the growing tensions between medicine, nursing and management illustrate

"Clear examples of irrational outcomes of growing rationalisation."

These tensions, in north America, have resulted in a situation in which:

"While the medical profession and health care administrators are attempting to expand the utilisation of technological devices in medicine, members of the nursing profession are striving to cope with their humanitarian consequences. Therefore nurses are trapped between two competing paradigms."

If we accept Hewa and Hetherington's (1990) notion that such a tension exists, then in nursing nowhere will the potential for this become more apparent than in the operation of Clinical Nurse Specialist roles. To date in the United Kingdom it has been the medical culture within which most posts have developed. Any occupational group which holds a monopoly over a particular area of work, as was granted to medicine under the 1858 Medical Act, has not only status, but also power (Wilding, 1982). Illich (1977) sees the medical profession as a 'monopolistic oligarchy' acting to determine needs which legally they alone can meet. The defining of need may not coincide with the consumers needs or wants, however a profession's ability to define need in the modern state ensures the perpetuation of the profession's influence on policy (Wilding, 1982; Friedson, 1970). This process will continue to propagate a medically defined concept of health, with a resulting organisation of services, such as the development of Clinical Nurse Specialist posts, in danger of being based on medically defined areas of practice, or professional skills, and not client need. This concern was echoed by the International Council of Nurses; (ICN) (1992) in their *Guidelines on 'Specialisation in Nursing'* who expressed concern that "developments may spin out of control, weakening the holistic nature of the profession."

The concern about Clinical Nurse Specialists operating under a proxy medical model was explored by Kerrison (1990) in her ethnographic study of the work of Diabetes Liaison Nurses. Following on the Weberian lines, the study explored how Doctors promoted the role of a Clinical Nurse Specialist as it allowed the delegation of 'psycho-social work' in which nurses claimed greater expertise. By taking on this work, nurses furthered their aspirations for professional status, while at the same time avoiding an open admission of taking over medical work, therefore avoiding an overt confrontation with the medical staff (Kerrison, 1990). This strategy of delegation could be seen as a means to ameliorate the tension

2

between the paradigms that Hewa and Hetherington (1990) described given the uncertain consequences of any confrontation. One possible consequence could be the withdrawal of support by the medical practitioner concerned. In such a case, unless the Clinical Nurse Specialist role is firmly rooted in nursing, it is probable that the viability of the role could be called into question (Kerrison, 1990).

This combination of forces serves to face Clinical Nurse Specialists with a potential dilemma. If the course of rational, instrumental choice continues then there will be a stage at which the value systems of nursing may be challenged. If the process is incremental it may not be fully apparent, however the organisational position of most Clinical Nurse Specialists places them at the forefront of any challenges on the values of nursing.

Clinical Nurse Specialist roles, therefore, lie somewhere between these two forces, both of which constantly vie to be the dominant influence. Clinical Nurse Specialists are at the mercy of the prevailing forces within wider society. These forces, such as rationalisation, or the medical model, may prove difficult to resist, especially as so many posts in the United Kingdom have been developed at the instigation of medical Consultants. However, the ICN (1992) has identified specialisation as "the path whereby nursing practice is deepened and refined," and this process has much to contribute to the changing nature of health care provision in the United Kingdom, which in turn may lead to a re-examination of legitimising boundaries of professional working (Kerrison, 1990). If this were to occur, it presents Clinical Nurse Specialists with an opportunity to demonstrate their worth, and to prosper professionally from such changes – while at the same time enabling them to grasp the opportunity that political and public recognition of the value of the role would bring (Hamric, 1992). Yet while there is an absence of official legitimation of such role changes, Clinical Nurse Specialists remain vulnerable to wider legal and professional processes.

The evidence of a shifting division of labour within nursing has been manifest in the increasing number of Clinical Nurse Specialist posts advertised in the nursing press. Bowman and Thompson (1990) illustrated the dangers of this rapid growth, suggesting that Nurse Specialists could be seen as medical assistants. The grave nature of this warning should not be underestimated, if professional nursing practice is to be valued. Clinical Nurse Specialist posts must be well defined in relation to the nursing role which they fulfil, but many posts remain ill-defined at the outset, as the concept of Nurse Specialism becomes elaborated in the light of experience in many organisations. This lack of clarity in itself can lead to a diminution of the role, as Nurse Specialists attempt to be

3

'all things to all people'. The danger of this scenario is that the Clinical Nurse Specialist then fails to fulfil any part of the role effectively (Malone, 1986), or burns out in the process of attempting to do so!

SPECIALITY AND SPECIALISM

It is important from the outset to explore and differentiate speciality from specialism. It could be argued that as soon as nurses qualify and work within a particular area of care that they are in a speciality, and therefore have started to specialise. So what stimulates specialities to develop? It is evident that in the United Kingdom the medical profession has traditionally exercised a very powerful influence over the shape of both the organisation and delivery of care. One consequence of this has been the appointment of nurses who are highly skilled in one area of work, and become specialists and as a consequence are able to exercise greater autonomy (Kerrison, 1990). For Papenhasen and Beecroft (1990) writing from a north American perspective, specialisation by nurses provides evidence of the advancement of the profession as a whole. Clearly, however, the issue of specialisation has been on the north American nursing agenda much longer than in the United Kingdom. Indeed, in 1980 the American Nurses' Association identified the factors which it considered precipitated specialisation. These included: an increasing amount and complexity of knowledge and technology; the need to obtain greater depth of understanding of a segment of nursing and to test new practices related to that segment of nursing; the centring of public attention and funds on an area of nursing practice; the complexity of services exceeding the prevailing knowledge and skills of the general practitioners; and the expansion of part of a professional field (Papenhausen and Beecroft, 1990).

In a similar attempt to add to the debate in the United Kingdom the Royal College of Nursing (1988) (RCN) citing the ICN (1986), suggested a range of factors which have influenced the development of "Specialities in Nursing". These included the need for a more effective use of the nurse workforce, changing sociological, cultural and economic factors affecting health care, advances in medical practice, the specific health-care needs of a population, and developing national priorities in health care (RCN, 1988). For the RCN (1988), a nursing speciality is seen as a component of the whole field of nursing, usually identified by being concerned with age, sex or population group, a body system, health status and even methods of investigation. While many Clinical Nurse Specialist roles are predominantly shaped by medically defined areas of practice, there are specialist roles which are emerging as a consequence of the expansion of nursing knowledge (Wright, 1992).

4

Therefore, can we, and where do we draw the line between speciality and specialism? Developments in speciality nurses appear not to have been planned in a particularly systematic way, and the development of nursing specialities has most often paralleled developments in medicine. So the need to differentiate between speciality nursing and specialism becomes more acute. Clearly the dominance of the medical model on the organisation and delivery of patient care in the United Kingdom has fundamentally influenced the development of nurse specialism, and Bowman and Thompson (1990) asserted this point in suggesting that:

"The problem with current 'nurse specialists' is that they develop in a system that organises its patients into groups convenient for medical strategies."

This was reiterated by the RCN (1988) in its document on 'specialities', in which the authors indicated that a considerable amount of the confusion about the nurse specialist role stems from the fact that there are many nurses in specialist posts who are not specialists, which is a concern expressed by a number of authors (Bowman and Thompson, 1990; Casey, 1990). These concerns have led to calls by Clinical Nurse Specialists for some form of direction and guidance, even regulation from the United Kingdom Central Council (UKCC), thus helping to ensure that Nurse Specialists remain firmly rooted in nursing. Guidance of this nature is clearly of enormous assistance to all concerned with the development and appointment of Clinical Nurse Specialists. And at the same time it helps to deal with the actual and potential problems of creating a new generation of doctors' handmaidens, by ensuring that Clinical Nurse Specialists are appropriately qualified to undertake their role. Bowman and Thompson (1990) are quite vehement in their view that "the title 'nurse specialist' should be reserved for those whose work is without doubt fixed in nursing."

WHAT MAKES A SPECIALIST?

Paralleled with medical developments, has clearly been the on-going development of nursing knowledge. At the same time, changes in the organisation of the National Health Service (NHS) have led to increased expectations of health care users. These factors, combined with a professional desire to constantly improve the quality of service delivery, will necessitate some form of formal qualification as a Clinical Nurse Specialist in order to ensure the protection of the public. In attempting to tackle this issue, the Canadian Nurses Association (1982) defined the characteristics of a Clinical Nurse Specialist, since a nurse "with advanced education and a research base is a natural concomitant to the expansion of knowledge."

Beecroft and Papenhausen (1988) suggest that

"the specialist is someone who is recognised and sought after by others because of advanced education in a particular area."

The ICN (1992) proposed that

"The nurse specialist is a nurse prepared beyond the level of a nurse generalist and authorised to practise as a specialist with advanced expertise in a branch of the nursing field. Speciality practice includes clinical, teaching, administration, research and consultant roles. Post-basic nursing education for speciality practice is a formally recognised programme of study built upon the general education for the nurse and providing the content and experience to ensure competency in speciality practice."

Specialists are, therefore experts in a particular area, or about the needs of a specific client group, with advanced education and a research base firmly rooted in nursing. These factors appear to represent the generic or core basis of specialist practice, which is common to all Clinical Nurse Specialists, and such generic factors could form the basis of a set of core competencies for all Clinical Nurse Specialists. If these were established it would provide a much greater opportunity for the effective evaluation and understanding of the role (Hamric and Spross, 1989).

The issue of the preparation for the role of Clinical Nurse Specialist was considered by Storr (1988) who examined the role as portrayed in the north American literature. From this work Storr (1988) suggested that it is imperative that the Clinical Nurse Specialist title be reserved for advanced practitioners, prepared, as in the United States of America, at Masters Degree level. Anything less, she suggests, will continue to result in confusion, for the inappropriate use of the title can lead to the potential dilution and misunderstanding of the role. While it is difficult to make direct cross-cultural translations, it would seem that the recommendations of Post Registration Education & Practice Project (UKCC, 1991) are inexorably moving the Clinical Nurse Specialist role towards graduate status. Indeed this movement is gaining sufficient momentum to become a natural consequence of securing a Clinical Nurse Specialist post. What is evident from the literature is that without appropriately advanced preparation for the role of a Clinical Nurse Specialist, complete role fulfilment will not be possible (Papenhausen and Beecroft,

1990). Moreover, given the constant evolution of the very factors put forward in the literature to explain the development of specialisation in nursing, and the necessary advanced preparation, we may well reach a point in the next century at which, as Moloney (1986) suggests, preparation for Clinical Nurse Specialisation at Masters Degree level may be the recognised "entry into practice" for professional nursing.

The three key characteristics, which from the literature act to define the Clinical Nurse Specialist are those of:

Graduate education
Practice based in research
Firm base as specialist in nursing

Given the degree of consensus on these broad characteristics of the individual Clinical Nurse Specialist, there is rather less consensus on the dimensions of the role. It is here that the application of role theory clearly has a contribution to make in the negotiation and construction of role definition statements. Such statements can act to identify the normative parameters of the role. The process of constructing a role statement requires a considerable degree of negotiation with the members identified within the Clinical Nurse Specialist role set. This process provides an opportunity to establish a wider and clearer understanding of the role with those with whom the Clinical Nurse Specialist interacts. Enhancing the wider understanding of the role will also assist in dealing with the dilemma of Clinical Nurse Specialists attempting to be 'all things to all people' (Hamric and Spross, 1989).

STAFF OR LINE POSITION

The position of the Clinical Nurse Specialist within the organisation of health care can also have a profound effect on the perception, and effectiveness, of the role. So should Clinical Nurse Specialists occupy a line or staff position? A staff position is defined as one in which the Clinical Nurse Specialist has no human resource management or budget responsibility, while the line position is one in which the Clinical Nurse Specialist is also a manager of the service and its resources.

The debate on this issue has been predominantly a north American one. However with the establishment of Clinical Directorates it is now becoming equally pertinent in the United Kingdom, as evidenced by the increasing number of advertisements for Clinical Nurse Specialists/ manager posts. Inherent in this situation is a dichotomy for the individual practitioner. In general, the literature makes the distinction between professional power associated with a staff position, and managerial power associated with a line position.

The Clinical Nurse Specialist in a staff position is said to rely on personal and professional power, the latter resulting from the individual's ability to achieve goals where others have failed to produce tangible results. Arguments in favour of the Clinical Nurse Specialist holding a staff position are threefold. Firstly, by holding a staff position they are less likely to be seen as a threat by other nursing staff, who then provide much needed support. Indeed it is suggested that in a staff position they actively increase productivity via the support they give, and so, it is suggested, improve the quality of care. A second reason to favour the Clinical Nurse Specialist holding a staff position is that the consultant and educator subroles are made easier if they are unencumbered by the managerial/administrational role. Finally, the managerial/administration function dilutes the specialist role and reduces visibility, which are two major components in improving the quality of care.

In opposition to this are the arguments that only Clinical Nurse Specialists in a line position, with the power to apply sanctions, can be effective agents of change. This allows them to augment their role by incorporating management principles, thus ensuring that the client receives the appropriate care from the appropriate staff. Finally it is suggested that the Clinical Nurse Specialists who have budgetary control can 'call the shots' and that only they can identify the appropriate services that can be delivered within the available resources. The moral and ethical dilemmas inherent in these positions are not explored to any great extent in the literature. Clearly no absolute conclusion can be reached, as it may be that the multi-dimensional nature of the Clinical Nurse Specialist role is both problem and solution.

In effect it is suggested that the Clinical Nurse Specialist in a line position, with a managerial component, is the preferred model. Yet this is often not the case and an excessive managerial load may be highlighted by a dilution of clinical expertise.

DEFINING THE ROLE

While there is a high degree of consensus on the broad characteristics of the individual Clinical Nurse Specialist, there is far less agreement on what constitutes the boundaries of the role. The use of role theory as a framework suggests that it is vital to have a clear definition of the role and its positioning within an organisation. A role definition statement is derived from the expectations of those members of the Clinical Nurse Specialist's role set.

Role theory is that which has as its domain of study real-life behaviour in a social environment. There are a number of stakeholders (Figure 1.1) who will all have varying expectations of a Clinical Nurse Specialist service, which may include colleagues, manager, service users and their representatives, service purchasers, as well as appropriate voluntary organisations (Morath, 1988). These differing parties clearly have a diverse range of expectations about the service, and such a situation clearly has the potential to generate considerable role conflict for individual Clinical Nurse Specialists. If a process of on-going dialogue with the role set members is established this will enable the parameters of the role to be clearly defined, rather than guessed. A role definition statement is therefore a combination of the expectations of those people within the Clinical Nurse Specialist's role set. These expectations may be occupationally, legally and professionally defined, and in turn set within the wider context of the health care system and society at large.

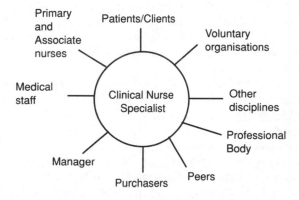

Figure 1.1 *Clinical Nurse Specialist role set*

Role theory focuses on the study of people and the roles they occupy. It provides a framework within which to explore the interactions and dynamics of the multiple roles an individual occupies at any one time (Handy, 1987). Within the literature on the role of the Clinical Nurse Specialist there are varying views on what constitutes the sub-roles, for Spross and Baggerley (1989) the role has both direct and indirect functions:

9

Direct	Indirect
Expert practitioner	Innovator
Role model	Change agent
Patient advocate	Consultant/Resource person
	Teacher
	Supervisor
	Researcher/Liaison

The RCN (1988) approached this issue from the perspective that only if nurses were involved in all the following areas could they claim to be specialists:

Clinical practice
Consultative role
Teaching
Management
Research and the application of research findings.

From the many examples in the literature of what constitutes the sub-roles of the Clinical Nurse Specialist, the majority appears to focus around the six sub-roles identified by Ryan-Merritt *et al.* (1988):

Director of care
Collaborator
Teacher
Educator
Researcher
Manager

For each of these six sub-roles it is possible to identify the behaviours and interventions appropriate to help operationalise that sub-role. The methodology adopted by Ryan-Merritt *et al.* (1988) was used as the basis of a learning contract in a Masters degree programme for Clinical Nurse Specialists. Students were able to use the framework as a series of competency statements to provide a basis to plan learning experiences. This approach includes the opportunity to formulate individualised objectives for self-development, and a basis for both formative and summative evaluation; as well as serving to illustrate the commonalties of Clinical Nurse Specialist practice. Utilising this framework, the following is an example of a role definition statement formulated by a Clinical Nurse Specialist working in a Department of Medicine for the Elderly.

Facilitator of learning

Identify educational needs of nursing staff in the Department of Medicine for the Elderly.
Provide and/or organise appropriate learning experiences to meet identified needs.
Evaluate the outcome of learning experiences with individual members of staff.
Initiate and provide individual orientation programmes for all nursing staff in the Department of Medicine for the Elderly.
Maintain accurate and up-to-date records of educational experiences of all nursing staff.
Liaise with the Department of Professional Development.

Provider of clinical care

Act as a role model in providing direct patient care.
Contribute to comprehensive patient assessments as appropriate.
Assist in developing plans of nursing care with the ward staff based on advanced clinical knowledge and expertise.
Provide direct nursing care on a regular basis.
Provide appropriate health education support and advice for patients and relatives.

Nursing care consultancy

Provide expert clinical nursing advice in relation to the care of elderly people.
Assess the need for consultation, collect and interpret information and prescribe action.
Provide support in carrying out the prescribed action.

Research

Evaluate research findings for implementation in practice.
Disseminate appropriate research findings with recommendations for practice.
Promote inquiry and evaluation of clinical practice.
Collaborate with other health care professionals in the development and implementation of research.
Act as an advocate to protect the rights of patients.

Collaborator

Work in co-operation with members of the multi-disciplinary team to benefit patient care.

Participate in multi-disciplinary groups.

Participate in the appointment of nursing staff.

Undertake other duties as negotiated with senior management.

Promoter of quality care

To be aware of and act in accordance with the policies, procedures and philosophy of the Health Authority.

To be aware of and adhere to the UKCC Code of Professional Conduct.

Facilitate and enable the implementation of the quality assurance programme in the Department of Medicine for the Elderly.

Serve as a member of the quality assurance committee for the Department of Medicine for the Elderly.

With such a framework is it possible to take a competency-based approach to the development of the individual practitioner within the role. Many of the competencies are generic, or core to all Clinical Nurse Specialist roles, while others are specific to the service that has been developed. However, no matter what the area of practice, if the role is inadequately defined it will result in evaluation beset with difficulties (Everson, 1981; Malone, 1986).

DANGERS AND DILEMMAS

The rapid growth in the number and range of Clinical Nurse Specialist posts is, for many, evidence of the unique contribution such a practitioner can make to the quality of nursing care. It has also been equated with the coming of age of the nursing profession, a sign of greater depth and rigour, with a breaking away from the traditional hierarchies (Altschul, 1982; Moloney, 1986; Beecroft and Papenhausen, 1987; American Nurses' Association, 1980; Wright, 1992). While such a display of professional unity provides a clear message about Nurse Specialism, the profession must remain mindful that the majority of nurses are not Specialists. The very same rapid growth in Clinical Nurse Specialists which so many writers applaud, and the moving away from medically dominated hierarchies, could result in the creation of similar structures within nursing. While Altschul (1982) asserts that generalists should not assume that theirs is the only and absolute truth, it would seem equally hazardous for

Clinical Nurse Specialists to assume that of themselves. Clearly while all nurses have a general knowledge base, the possession of specialist knowledge and skills will be held by fewer members of the profession (Chisholm, 1991). Clinical Nurse Specialists therefore could be said to know more and more about less and less (Wade and Moyer, 1989). Although the vast expansion of nursing knowledge necessitates this situation, there is the danger of fragmentation in both accountability and continuity (Sparacino, 1991). Indeed the ICN (1992) warns of the possible fragmentation of nursing care if Clinical Nurse Specialism develops in a 'disorderly' pattern. The obvious question that follows is: 'At what point does the intervention of a number of Clinical Nurse Specialists, called upon by the named primary nurse, to participate in an individual's care, become task allocation by another name?'. In a similar vein, Salvage (1985) warned that nurses tend to accept, uncritically, that professionalisation has only positive ramifications, while ignoring the negative effects, such as the potential for divisiveness (Jolley, 1989). The development of specialisation within work processes has resulted in a considerable body of work related to the concept of deskilling (Storch and Stinson, 1988). One of the major contributors to this field of work is Braverman (1974) who suggests that the labour process is shaped by the provision of labour power as cheaply as possible. If this is considered within the context of the clinical grading of most Nurse Specialists, clearly there are resource planning issues which need to be addressed if a career structure is to be sustainable. An additional dilemma lies within the relationship between the Clinical Nurse Specialist and the primary nurse. The Clinical Nurse Specialist directs the primary nurse about the precise care which should be delivered in a specific situation and this situation becomes compounded as the range of Clinical Nurse Specialists increases, thus creating a situation in which generalists may abdicate various aspects of care. This has the potential to create a damaging schism within the profession resulting in the establishment of an elite. Clinical Nurse Specialists must be mindful of the need for a mutual partnership for the ultimate benefit of the recipients of care.

CONCLUSION

The complex organisations within which Clinical Nurse Specialists work exert an elaborate range of pressures and expectations on them. The massive growth in the number and range of Clinical Nurse Specialists has economic considerations within an increasingly, financially scrutinised system (Gift, 1992; Nugent, 1992). Specialisation is a natural progression within nursing, and so it will continue, and therefore changes in the Clinical Nurse Specialist role are inevitable. Wider pressures within health care necessitate evidence of the effectiveness of the role, and failure to define the role will make it difficult to gather valid and reliable evidence (Everson, 1981). The use of role theory provides the Clinical Nurse Specialist with a framework for the generation and progression of the role. Such an approach, with its process of negotiation, ensures that the evolving role remains sensitive to the needs and expectations of those within the Clinical Nurse Specialist's role set. While Clinical Nurse Specialists clearly make a very valuable, necessary contribution to the care of individuals, and to the development of the nursing profession as a whole, there are potential dangers associated with such developments. It is vital that Clinical Nurse Specialists remain alert to the dangers and continue to enhance mutual partnerships with professional colleagues which benefit those for whom the service exists, namely, the consumer.

REFERENCES

Altschul A. (1982) Specifics and rigour. *Nursing Mirror*, September 1, p. 27.

American Nurses' Association (1980) *Nursing: A Social Policy Statement.* ANA, Kansas City.

Beecroft P.C. and Papenhausen J.L. (1987) Editorial opinion. *Clinical Nurse Specialist*, 1(1): 1.

Beecroft P.C. and Papenhausen J.L. (1988) What is a specialist? *Clinical Nurse Specialist*, 2(3): 109–112.

Bowman G. and Thompson P. (1990) When is a specialist not a specialist? *Nursing Times*, 86(8): 48.

Braverman H. (1974) *Labour and Monopoly Capitalism.* Monthly Review Press, New York.

Canadian Nurses Association (1982) *Credentialing in Nursing: Policy Statement and Background Paper.* Canadian Nurses Association, Ottawa.

Casey N. (1990) The specialist debate. *Nursing Standard*, 4(3): 18–19.

Chisholm M. (1991) Collaboration: impacting professionalism and quality of care. *Clinical Nurse Specialist*, 5(4): 217.

Everson S.A. (1981) Integration of the role of the Clinical Nurse Specialist. *Journal of Continuing Education in Nursing*, 12(2): 16–19.

Friedson E. (1970) *Professional Powers: A Study of the Institutionalization of Formal Knowledge.* University of Chicago Press, Chicago, Illinois.

Gift A.G. (1992) Determining CNS cost effectiveness. *Clinical Nurse Specialist*, 6(2): 89.

Hamric A. (1992) Resolving the health care crisis: where is the CNS? *Clinical Nurse Specialist*, 6(2): 105.

Hamric A. and Spross J. (1989) *The Clinical Nurse Specialist in Theory and Practice*, 2nd edn. Saunders, Philadelphia, Pennsylvania.

Handy C.B. (1987) *Understanding Organisations*, 3rd edn. Penguin, Harmondsworth, Middlesex.

Hewa S. and Hetherington R. (1990) Specialists without spirit: crisis in the nursing profession. *Journal of Medical Ethics*, 16: 179–184.

Illich I. (1977) *Disabling Professions*. Boyars, London.

International Council of Nurses (1986) Professional Services Committee: Specialisation in Nursing, Revised draft ICN/86/148. In *Specialities in Nursing*. Royal College of Nursing, London.

International Council of Nurses (1992) *Guidelines on 'Specialisation in Nursing'*. ICN, Geneva.

Jolley, M. (1989) The professionalisation of nursing: the uncertain path. In Jolley M. and Allan P. (Eds), *Current Issues in Nursing*. Chapman and Hall, London.

Kerrison S. (1990) *A Diplomat in the Job: Diabetes Nursing and the Changing Division of Labour in Diabetic Care*. Research Paper 4, Health & Social Services Research Unit, South Bank Polytechnic, London.

Lane B. (1985) Specialisation in nursing: some Canadian issues. *Canadian Nurse*, June 24–25.

Malone B. (1986) Working with people: evaluation of the Clinical Nurse Specialist. *American Journal of Nursing*, 86(12): 1375–1377.

Moloney M.M. (1986) *Professionalization of Nursing Current Issues and Trends*. Lippincott, Philadelphia, Pennsylvania.

Morath J. (1988) The CNS: evaluation issues. *Nursing Management*, 19(3): 72–80.

Nugent K.E. (1992) The Clinical Nurse Specialist as case manager in a collaborative practice model: bridging the gap between quality and cost of care. *Clinical Nurse Specialist*, 6(2): 106–111.

Papenhausen J.L and Beecroft P.C. (1990) Specialization vis-a-vis the Clinical Nurse Specialist. *Clinical Nurse Specialist*, 4(2): 61–62.

Royal College of Nursing (1988) *Specialities in Nursing*. Royal College of Nursing, London.

Ryan-Merritt V.M., Mitchell C.A. and Pagel I. (1988) Clinical Nurse Specialist role definition and operationalization. *Clinical Nurse Specialist*, 2(3): 132–137.

Salvage J. (1985) *The Politics of Nursing*. Heinemann Nursing, London.

Sparacino P.S. (1991) The CNS–case manager relationship. *Clinical Nurse Specialist*, 5(4): 180–181.

Spross J.A. and Baggerley J. (1989) Models of advanced nursing practice. In Hamric A. and Spross J. (1989).

Storch J.L. and Stinson S.M. (1988) Concepts of deprofessionalisation with applications to nursing. In White R. (Ed.), *Political Issues in Nursing Vol. 3*. Wiley, Chichester.

Storr G. (1988) The Clinical Nurse Specialist from the outside looking in. *Journal of Advanced Nursing*, 13(2): 265–272.

United Kingdom Central Council for Nursing, Midwifery and Health Visiting (1991) *Post Registration Education & Practice Project*. UKCC, London.

Wade B. and Moyer A. (1989) An evaluation of clinical nurse specialists: implications for education and the organisation of care. *Senior Nurse*, 9(9): 11–16.

Wilding P. (1982) *Professional Power and Social Welfare*. Routledge and Kegan Paul, London.

Wright S.G. (1992) Advances in clinical practice. *British Journal of Nursing*, 1(4): 192.

CHAPTER TWO

Models of specialist practice

Fiona Cameron

The aim of this chapter is to explore differing models and frameworks which may be utilised by the nurse specialist in organising and operationalising the role. Fundamental to this exploration is some discussion aimed at explicating the differences between theoretical and conceptual models. Existing models or frameworks will be outlined and their merits discussed in relation, not only to their ability to direct practice, but their ability to guide nurses in the search for nursing theory. Utilising the role definition statement from Chapter 1 the roles of the Clinical Nurse Specialist will be related to practice with particular emphasis on the Clinical Nurse Specialist as direct care giver. Those factors impacting on the Clinical Nurse Specialist in this role will be outlined and survival strategies discussed. The importance of being explicit regarding the utilisation of a conceptual model of practice to explicate the Clinical Nurse Specialist role and to expand the body of knowledge that is uniquely nursing will be illuminated.

MODELS AND THEORIES – A DISTINCTION

A discussion on theory may seem at best an accumulation of words to increase the academic vocabulary. However a basic understanding of the difference between theory and conceptual models is central to this chapter. Indeed this chapter will show that without the above understanding, progression of the Clinical Nurse Specialist role will be self limiting.

'Theory' according to Riehl and Roy (1980), is a "logically interconnected set of propositions used to describe explain and predict a part of the empirical world." In other words theory will rationalise and delimit a particular phenomena. A 'model', on the other hand, "is a conceptual

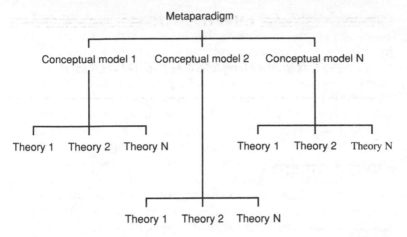

Figure 2.1   *The structural hierarchy of knowledge (Fawcett, 1984)*

representation of reality" (Riehl and Roy, 1980). The difference between a model and a theory lies in the level of abstraction attributable.

Fawcett (1984), illuminates this distinction in the following way:

" a conceptual model is a highly abstract system of global concepts and propositions."

" a theory deals with one or more specific, concrete concepts and propositions."

Theory quite simply enables the operationalisation of a given conceptual model. Viewed in this way the utility of the use of conceptual models in nurse specialist practice needs little support. Figure 2.1 is a diagrammatic representation of the structural hierarchy of knowledge and serves to illuminate this point.

The metaparadigm phenomena of nursing, person, health and environment are generally accepted as the components addressed by nursing theory (Riehl and Roy, 1980; Fawcett, 1984). Therefore a single metaparadigm may be represented conceptually in a number of ways and illuminated via a range of theories.

There is some argument in the literature as to the necessity of the metaparadigm nursing, in nursing theory construction, and theories whose derivation is from the combination of the metaparadigm phenomena of nursing, person, health and environment are considered to be more encompassing and sophisticated. However theories derived from any of the metaparadigm phenomena can be considered as nursing theories provided they are bound up in the context of nursing.

Theories are classified as descriptive, explanatory and predictive and constructed via inductive, deductive and retroductive methods. In the deductive mode of enquiry, theory construction commences with a set of propositions which may be tested to confirm or deny their truth. Theory is deduced from the testing of a given hypothesis. In inductive theory the hypothesis is induced. That is to say, the theorist commences with a number of concepts or a general orientation and searches for their meaning and relatedness in a particular setting. Retroductive methods combine both deduction and induction to build theory.

Debate regarding the utility of these methods of theory construction is to be found in the nursing literature, particularly in relation to qualitative and quantitative approaches to research. Two competing paradigms are associated with qualitative and quantitative approaches with the inductive method aligning itself with qualitative approaches and the deductive method with quantitative. The paradigm assumptions underpinning these, of *human science* and *scientific method*, have had a significant effect on nursing research and theory construction. The literature abounds with accounts of nurses' predilection with the scientific method, relating it to the process of professionalisation and status; while many argue that the very nature of nursing ties it to more human science approaches and methods. This debate notwithstanding, there is considerable pressure upon nurses to utilise integrated approaches to theory construction. However, the choice of a conceptual model of practice will at least, to some degree, determine the route taken in the theory construction process.

CONCEPTUAL MODELS – A SELECTION

"In nursing, conceptual models are used as general guides for organisation of nursing knowledge and the design and implementation of nursing practice."

Fawcett (1984)

Given the above it is reasonable to expect a conceptual model of practice to guide nurse education, nursing research, nursing administration and nursing practice. So, what is a model of specialist practice?

A model of specialist practice must guide clinical practice, education, research and administration in much the same way as other conceptual models of practice and is therefore of necessity compatible with the orientation of the model or models in use in any given area. More important however, suggest Spross and Baggerly (1989), is the ability of the conceptual model to illuminate the concepts of clinical judgement and leadership. The rationale for this observation is rooted in the assumption that Clinical Nurse Specialists exercise both judgement at an advanced level and leadership relating not only to practice development but strategically in relation to finance, research and education.

Hamric and Spross (1989), provide a clear description of a range of models of specialist practice and it is not the aim of this chapter to redefine them. However three models will be described, with emphasis on their proactivity and utility in relation to Clinical Nurse Specialist practice. There are significant differences between the models chosen and this is deliberate, as the usefulness of any model of practice lies in its ability to guide without prescription and work in the setting. There are however, some similarities, for each model has, as its focus, direct care provision and is explicit regarding the advanced judgement required of the Clinical Nurse Specialist and the notion of leadership.

CASE MANAGEMENT MODEL

Papenhausen (1990) proposes Case Management as a model for advanced practice which, utilised by the Clinical Nurse Specialist, offers a cost-effective use of resource in a clearly defined practice arena. Case Management is defined by Papenhausen (1990) as a vehicle for providing care which is balanced in terms of cost and quality. A distinction is made between the terms *managed care* and *case management*, the latter being associated with greater personalised interaction between the client and the case manager. A number of models of case management are available (Papenhausen, 1990; Sinnen and Schifalacqua, 1991), variously entitled

- the acute care model;
- the Arizona model;
- the health maintenance model;
- the public health model;
- the nursing centre model.

The commonalty in these models lies in their having the client as the central focus and their progression through a number of fixed points: client entry – predictive phase – client exit.

These models focus on specific client groups and identify clearly at which point clients become the focus of the model, for example, utilising the public health model the Clinical Nurse Specialist would see all clients presenting with special needs. The Clinical Nurse Specialist is viewed as having the intellectual ability, clinical competence and strategic orientation to provide client-centred quality care which takes account of cost

19

while retaining efficacy and individuality. Clients enter the system of case management by virtue of their specificity. Utilising a case management model the Clinical Nurse Specialist with advanced practice skills predicts the outcome of intervention for each individual in terms of cost, quality, optimal achievement level and in a holistic manner.

The utilisation of this model with specific client groups, and in particular those client groups who are viewed as expensive in terms of health care, is supported by Papenhausen (1990). This model has obvious merit in relation to Clinical Nurse Specialist practice with specific client groups such as those with AIDS, specific psychiatric conditions and learning disabilities. However, the orientation of the model is such that except for a very few areas, autonomous practice of this nature for Clinical Nurse Specialist is futuristic. However, the current trend toward care management arising from the documents, 'Caring for People' and 'Working for Patients' is a step in this direction which may well spread as community care becomes a reality in the mid 1990s.

This model can be seen to meet the needs of the client group, enabling the Clinical Nurse Specialist to exercise expert judgement. The Leadership role of the Clinical Nurse Specialist would, however, be necessarily curtailed within the client group and mechanisms of peer support and organisational interfacing needed to raise the role to a strategic level over a more global site. From a research perspective, the Clinical Nurse Specialist utilising this model is in a prime position to inform practice inductively.

INTERNAL CONSULTATION

The internal consultation framework for specialist practice is outlined by Noll (1987) and has as its focus, change agency and problem solving. This framework discusses consultancy in terms of internal and external, and postulates that Clinical Nurse Specialists can operationalise their role via internal consultations due to expert orientation and constancy of availability within a given organisation. Noll (1987) cites the rationale for employing an internal consultant as being the desire to enhance organisational development and outcomes. Given the above, few Clinical Nurse Specialists would argue that this model might have applicability.

The Clinical Nurse Specialist as internal consultant can be viewed as operating on a number of planes, consulted by patients, staff, management and other disciplines. The purpose of these consultations, one assumes, is based in problem solving and change facilitation, incorporating the sub-roles of practice, education and research. Thus the internal consultant Clinical Nurse Specialists operationalise their role, as direct care giver, co-ordinator of multi-disciplinary teams, policy maker, patient teacher, staff educator, research project leader, product evaluator and community resource.

Although there is no direct mention of the Clinical Nurse Specialist providing advanced judgement skills, these can be seen to be implicit in the operationalisation of the role. Noll (1987) does not offer any practical suggestions as to how the role might be implemented as the article is based on the organisation appointing a Clinical Nurse Specialist as internal consultant. If the Clinical Nurse Specialist wanted to utilise this framework, considerable negotiation with management and colleagues would have to take place before adopting this strategy. The model does however, have two significant advantages. The first is that the role can be seen to meet the demands of the client group, provided the referral criteria are consumer led. Secondly, this model can be viewed as lifting the Clinical Nurse Specialist role out of the nursing milieu, while retaining nursing at its core.

The research role of the Clinical Nurse Specialist can be viewed as one in which research is implemented as a means of evaluating outcomes of nursing intervention. One can assume from this that the research role has as its focus, the development of nursing theory from nursing practice issues. Certainly the outcome specific nature of this model of practice has merit in today's environment.

THE WORK OF BENNER AND FENTON

Spross and Baggerly (1989) combine Benner's (1984) work on clinical expertise and Fenton's (1985) further application of this to Clinical Nurse Specialist practice and suggest that the combination provides a useful model of advanced practice. The utility of this model is in the application of the domains of nursing:

● the helping role;
● administration and monitoring therapeutic interventions and regimes;
● effective management of rapidly changing situations;
● the diagnostic and monitoring functions;
● the teaching/coaching function;
● monitoring and ensuring the quality of health-care practices;
● organisational and work role competencies;
● the consulting role.

to the roles of the CNS.

The work of Benner (1984) and Fenton (1985) is extensively quoted in the nursing literature on Clinical Nurse Specialist role implementation

(Ryan-Merritt *et al.*, 1988; Storr, 1988; Hamric and Spross, 1989; Shawler *et al.*, 1990; Sparacino, 1990). The major benefit of utilising this model is deemed as its ability to define the role of the Clinical Nurse Specialist and accurately reflect its effect. The model is operationalised via the roles of the practitioner, educator, consultant and researcher and is viewed as addressing both clinical judgement and leadership.

Clinical judgement is exemplified in the model via its clear delineation of the skills involved while leadership is viewed as implicit in many of the competencies of the domains. The model can be seen to exhibit two distinct attributes which Clinical Nurse Specialists can harness in the development of their role. The emphasis on clinical practice, through the medium of expert clinical judgement, supports and maintains the uniqueness of nursing. However, this emphasis also raises the role to a level of functioning whose view offers strategic opportunities for developing the image and impact of nursing. The second attribute is the suggested way in which Clinical Nurse Specialists operationalise the research role. The model encourages the Clinical Nurse Specialist to employ reflection in practice strategies, to capture knowledge that is uniquely part of nursing and to inform practice through clinical ethnography. It is in this area, in particular, that further work might develop this model so that its utility for Clinical Nurse Specialists in the research role could be developed.

Models of specialist practice must, according to Hamric and Waterman Taylor (1989), have the ability to meet the changes which, of necessity, affect the role. That change is implicit in all Clinical Nurse Specialist practice is due to societal institutional and client group changing expectations. Benner (1984) identified change agency as one of the domains. Subsequently work by both Ryan-Merritt *et al.* (1988) and Hamric and Spross (1989) has placed the activity of change agent within each of the roles of the Clinical Nurse Specialist.

The model is flexible and can be utilised by a range of Clinical Nurse Specialists in different settings while retaining its flexibility. The model offers a very useful means of explaining the Clinical Nurse Specialist role to others as well as a vehicle for making explicit the integrative nature of the roles. The roles viewed in this way can offer the Clinical Nurse Specialist the opportunity to weight the roles to meet the ever changing needs of the client group, institution and staff. The model offers the Clinical Nurse Specialist a framework for evaluating the effectiveness of the role and once understood by other staff can be a means of eliciting feedback on staff perceptions of the role. The roles broken down into component parts can be a useful means of asking the question, am I doing this? Not only is feedback elicited on role success

22

for staff, but the Clinical Nurse Specialist can identify where the role needs to alter to meet staff needs.

The model has application in the real world. It clearly states what the Clinical Nurse Specialist does and does not do and can support any given model of nursing practice utilised by staff in the provision of nursing care. The model also offers a method of operationalising and lending weight to the research role with its emphasis on reflection in practice. There is considerable support in the literature in relation to this approach to generating research questions in nursing. Sparacino (1990) suggests that Clinical Nurse Specialists have a responsibility to actively pursue the research component of their role in the practice arena to influence theory development and refinement. The Clinical Nurse Specialist enables both the translation of theory in practice and practice to feed the development of theory. Murphy and Hoeffer (1983) identify the integrated nature of practice-generated theory and theory-based practice, and support the utility of the above in theory refinement.

THE DIRECT CARE SUB-ROLE

The importance of the direct care role cannot be overstated and is evidenced in the model's outlines. Even in the early stages of role development Page and Arena (1991) note the necessity of scheduling time for direct care activities and keeping that time sacrosanct. It is also of note that strategies are suggested for obtaining acceptance of the Clinical Nurse Specialist in this role including:

- wearing similar attire to other nurses;
- answering patient call bells; and
- working shifts.

(Hamric and Spross, 1989; Page and Arena, 1991)

While there is support for the premise that the role of the Clinical Nurse Specialist hinges on the direct care role, caution should be exercised when utilising the above strategies. Acceptance and credibility are essential to the role development and may not be attained by merging with the general milieu, otherwise the question might be asked – what makes the Clinical Nurse Specialist different from the experience practitioner?

Much of the referenced material in this chapter relates to north America and assumes the CNS to be prepared at Masters level. While it is not the purpose in this chapter to discuss the educational preparation of the Clinical Nurse Specialist the distinctions in this country deserve mention:

23

'The successful CNS is one who maintains clinical care as a primary focus, continues to excel in practice skills and articulates and demonstrates how advanced practice makes a difference'

Sparacino (1990)

If one can accept the above as true, then it could be suggested that making explicit the differences may be a successful route to acceptance and credibility. However, answering patient call bells and working on shifts are activities which do more than make the Clinical Nurse Specialist appear one of the team. Gaining acceptance and credibility can be easier to achieve than one might assume. Kramer (1974) suggested that new nurses are continually tested and Page and Arena (1991) postulate this to be the case with Clinical Nurse Specialists new to their role, or experienced Clinical Nurse Specialists new to the setting. This view has merit and can be related to the allocation of the patient perceived as 'difficult' to the Clinical Nurse Specialist. Hamric and Spross (1989) evidence the difficult or problem patient as a means of role modelling and staff development for the Clinical Nurse Specialist in the direct care role. The above is undoubtedly true, but grasping these opportunities amid cries from other nurses regarding time constraints and budgeting concerns can do much to enable the Clinical Nurse Specialist to be viewed as useful, and credible. Acceptance must surely follow. However there are dangers inherent in survival strategies which are driven by others. The Clinical Nurse Specialist must constantly guard against the expectations of staff driving and shaping the role to meet immediate short-term needs.

Time scheduled for direct patient care is suggested by Shawler *et al.* (1990) as the linchpin of the Clinical Nurse Specialist role. The importance of the direct care role is also evidenced by Sisson (1987) who identified that staff often felt the Clinical Nurse Specialist should do more of it. However, implementing the role of direct care is easier for some Clinical Nurse Specialists than others. A number of nurse specialists are population specific, however, there are dangers in the caseload strategy if patients seen by the Clinical Nurse Specialist are not markedly different from those seen by other practitioners or do not evidence different outcomes.

Hamric and Spross (1989) make a useful distinction between the unit-based and population-based Clinical Nurse Specialist. The unit-based Clinical Nurse Specialist is employed in one department or area, for example a Clinical Nurse Specialist in a Department of Medicine for the Elderly. The direct care role is evidenced via the care planning process and referral to the Clinical Nurse Specialist could be made by all disci-

Table 2.1 *Advantages and disadvantages of both unit-based and population-based Clinical Nurse Specialist (Hamic and Spross, 1989)*

Unit-based		Population-based	
Advantages	*Disadvantages*	*Advantages*	*Disadvantages*
Increased visibility	Limited environment	Developing institution-wide standards	Attempting to be all things to all people
Part of a defined team	Risk of inappropriate use	Less constraint from unit policies	Working in different sub-systems
Increased ability to evaluate role	Risk of members of client group in other areas not being seen	All patients with a given diagnosis seen – not reliant on referral systems	Expertise too dilute

plines within the Department. The population based Clinical Nurse Specialist, for example a Stoma Nurse Specialist, is employed by the larger organisation, a hospital or group of hospitals. The direct care role is evidenced via contact and documentation of this for every patient with a stoma referral is automatic. Table 2.1 highlights the advantages and disadvantages of both approaches.

In a ward setting the Clinical Nurse Specialist must make explicit rationales for direct patient care in terms of the benefits to the client/patient via documentation of patient care and interaction and partnerships with other disciplines which are outcome specific. Hamric and Spross (1989) allude to direct patient care as having a number of components encompassing assessment, planning, evaluation, advocacy and role modelling. However, the Clinical Nurse Specialist role in direct patient care cannot be viewed in isolation, other components of the role can and should be made explicit to staff while the Clinical Nurse Specialist practises direct care. Scheduled direct patient care by the Clinical Nurse Specialist enables collaboration, teaching, consulting, researching and quality issues to be illuminated.

It can be contended that direct care provision is central to the role as it enables exemplification and acceptance of all other roles assumed by the

Clinical Nurse Specialist. In a large department the lone Clinical Nurse Specialist may find direct care provision in all areas an impossible task and could fall into the trap of trying to be everywhere at once and all things to all people, thus diminishing the more strategic planning and leadership areas of the role. The temptation to be visible to everyone at once may be strong. However, giving in to this urge could render the Clinical Nurse Specialist a physical wreck at best and a dabbler at worst.

At this juncture it may be useful to choose a channel of least resistance. The areas/wards most in need of Clinical Nurse Specialist input may by their very nature be most resistant to interference. Consequently, starting in one area with an identified 'problem patient' or at the invitation of staff has a number of merits. Success, helpfulness, non-threatening support, once engendered, will be credited to you and as credibility of the role increases so pressure among ward managers increases to utilise the skills of the Clinical Nurse Specialist. Most Clinical Nurse Specialists will identify with the feeling of exhilaration of 'having arrived' associated with the telephone call from Ward 1 requesting assistance in the selection of, for instance, a pressure area support system/an appropriate assessment method or technique for hydrating a client.

Having outlined the centrality of the direct care component of the Clinical Nurse Specialist role, some discussion of the weighting attributable to the components of the role of the Clinical Nurse Specialist is necessary. Pollock (1987) has identified the poor attention paid to the research component, in addition there can be debate regarding the balance of teaching aimed at clients and nurses (Hamric and Spross, 1989). Unless the Clinical Nurse Specialist is explicit at the outset regarding both defining their role and operationalising it, any attempt to weight the roles will be lost in their intrinsic tendency to overlap. If one can achieve a clear role definition it should embrace the following:

- provide clinical care;
- provide specialist nursing advice;
- facilitate learning – patients;
- facilitate learning – staff;
- promote quality care;
- contribute to research;
- collaboration with others.

This explicit delineation of role components enables evaluation of the role, even when there is considerable overlap.

Being explicit in role definition about the sub-roles by separating them out in the form suggested by Ryan Merritt *et al.* (1988) enables the

Clinical Nurse Specialist to break the role down and evaluatively re-shape it to meet the needs of the client group both patient and staff. The distinction between what is theory and its relationship to conceptual models has been explored. Three conceptual models of practice for Clinical Nurse Specialists have been outlined with emphasis on the centrality of the direct care role. Finally the problems of operationalising the direct care sub-role have been discussed and related to a model of practice which enhances explicitness of the Clinical Nurse Specialist role. On a lighter note McCaffrey (1991) outlines the unspoken sub-roles of the Clinical Nurse Specialist which are both entertaining and evidence of the level of expectation of the role.

A conceptual model is essential, therefore, if the Clinical Nurse Specialist is to firstly survive, and secondly secure a base for practice which is firmly rooted in nursing.

REFERENCES

Benner P. (1984) *From Novice to Expert: Excellence and Power in Clinical Nursing Practice*. Addison-Wesley, Menlo Park, California.

Fawcett J. (1984) *Analysis and Evaluation of Conceptual Models of Nursing*. Davies, Philadelphia, Pennsylvania.

Fenton M.V. (1985) Identifying competences of clinical nurse specialists. *Journal of Nursing Administration,* 15(12): 31–37.

Hamric A.B. and Spross J.A. (1989) *The Clinical Nurse Specialist in Theory and Practice,* 2nd edn. Saunders, Philadelphia, Pennsylvania.

Hamric A. and Waterman Taylor J. (1989) Role development of the CNS. In Hamric A. and Spross J. (1989).

Kramer M. (1974) *Reality Shock: Why Nurses Leave Nursing*. Mosby, St. Louis, Missouri.

McCaffrey D. (1991) The unspoken sub-roles of the Clinical Nurse Specialist. *Clinical Nurse Specialist,* 5(2): 71–72.

Murphy J. and Hoeffer B. (1983) Role of the specialist in nursing science. *Advances in Nursing Science,* 5(4): 31–39.

Noll M.L. (1987) Internal consultation as a framework for CNS practice. *Clinical Nurse Specialist,* 1(1): 46–50.

Page N.E. and Arena D.M. (1991) Practical strategies for Clinical Nurse Specialist role implementation. *Clinical Nurse Specialist,* 5(1): 43–48.

Papenhausen J.L. (1990) Case Management: a model of advanced practice. *Clinical Nurse Specialist,* 4(4): 169–170.

Pollock S.E. (1987) Clinical nursing research: the needed link for unifying professional nursing. *Clinical Nurse Specialist,* 1(1): 8–12.

Riehl J. and Roy C. (1980) *Conceptual Models for Nursing Practice,* 2nd edn. Appleton-Century-Crofts, New York.

Ryan-Merritt M.V., Mitchell C.A. and Pagel I. (1988) Clinical Nurse Specialist role definition and operationalization. *Clinical Nurse Specialist*, 2(3): 132–137.

Shawler C., Stepler H. and Kinnaird S.W. (1990) Model for integration of Clinical Nurse Specialist with nursing management and staff development. *Clinical Nurse Specialist*, 4(2): 98–102.

Sinnen M.T. and Schifalacqua M.M. (1991) Co-ordinated care in a community hospital. *Nursing Management*, 22(3): 38–42.

Sisson R. (1987) Co-workers perception of the Clinical Nurse Specialist role. *Clinical Nurse Specialist*, 1(1): 13–17.

Sparacino P.S.A. (1990) Strategies for implementing advanced practice. *Clinical Nurse Specialist*, 4(3): 151–152.

Spross J.A. and Baggerly J. (1989) Models of advanced nursing practice. In Hamric A.B. and Spross J.A., *The Clinical Nurse Specialist in Theory and Practice*, 2nd edn. Saunders, Philadelphia, Pennsylvania.

Storr G. (1988) The CNS from the outside looking in. *Journal of Advanced Nursing*, 13(2): 265–272.

CHAPTER THREE

Research: motivator or generator?

Sheila Mackie Bailey

INTRODUCTION

Nursing research is research into those aspects of professional activity which are predominantly and appropriately the concern and responsibility of nurses (Cormack, 1984). The Clinical Nurse Specialist is in an ideal position to change and influence clinical practice and professional activity. The Clinical Nurse Specialist may choose to be involved in research, be an informed user of research, a disseminator of research findings or a promoter of research – all of which are essential to ensuring a high standard of patient care. Florence Nightingale is accredited with being the founder of modern nursing, but she also has the reputation of being the first nurse researcher of modern times. She earned this reputation because she was assiduous in the collection of facts to support her arguments for improvements in the care of people both in hospital and in the community. Thus she set a good example for today's Clinical Nurse Specialists; she was fearless in the pursuit of her ideas, values and beliefs, and having established the facts she argued vehemently for the changes she believed were necessary. Today's Clinical Nurse Specialists face the same challenge. In order to improve the quality of care their patients receive they must ensure that they themselves are well informed of the research developments which could affect their area of nursing practice. This has far reaching implications for Clinical Nurse Specialists as it must include not only those aspects of clinical practice which are particular to their specialty but all aspects of the care their patients receive, and it requires that the Clinical Nurse Specialist adopts a holistic, not a blinkered, approach to care delivery. Do today's Clinical Nurse Specialists have the courage and integrity of Florence Nightingale?

In order to meet these standards of performance it requires that today's Clinical Nurse Specialists must ensure that their practice is beyond reproach, and meet, if not excel, the standard which the United Kingdom Central Council (UKCC) sets for all qualified nurses in the *Code of Professional Conduct* (1992). The current edition of the Code includes an important change of emphasis. It states that:

> "As a registered nurse, midwife or health visitor you are personally accountable for your practice and, in the exercise of your professional accountability, **must**..."

The shift in emphasis from 'should' to 'must' is significant. Relevant to this discussion the *Code of Professional Conduct* (1992) states that you **must**

> "maintain and improve your professional knowledge and competence"

This is a challenging statement for nurses, midwives and health visitors, but especially for the Clinical Nurse Specialist who must be knowledgeable and competent in two respects: as a general practitioner and as a specialist. This makes a research base for practice imperative.

BACKGROUND

Despite the example set by Florence Nightingale it was the late 1950s before nursing research in the United Kingdom (UK) attracted the attention of 'curious' nurses, nurses who were concerned about improving the quality of care their patients received. One of the best known of those early researchers was Doreen Norton – her pressure sore risk assessment scale (Norton *et al.*, 1962), which she developed from her original research, has certainly stood the test of time. In the late 1950s and early 1960s Doreen Norton was a member of a small group of nurse researchers who banded together to provide each other with help and support. They formed the London based 'Research Discussion Group', which in the beginning was so small in membership that they met in each others' homes. Eventually the group became a membership group, the Research Society of the Royal College of Nursing (RCN), now the Research Advisory Group. Like the Research Discussion Group the function of both these groups is to provide nurse researchers with support and to promote the dissemination and utilisation of research findings.

The next milestone was the publication in 1972 of the 'Report of the Committee on Nursing', better known as the Briggs Report. The Report stated that "nursing must become a research based profession" though it qualified this statement by explaining that this did not mean that all nurses should become researchers. It took a further seven years for the

Report to be enacted by Parliament, and the profession, especially nurse educators, has been even slower to respond to this exhortation (Burnard and Chapman, 1990). However, in recent years there has been an increase in the amount of research undertaken by nurses, though the quality of such research has varied enormously and one of the challenges for the Clinical Nurse Specialist is to be able to distinguish between research findings which can be utilised, adopted into practice and those which are small-scale projects which do not meet the standards of *bona fide* research. To make such a judgement the Clinical Nurse Specialist needs to have an understanding of the main purposes of research in nursing, the stages of the research process, how to read a research report critically, and how to implement changes in nursing practice based upon research findings.

THE MAIN PURPOSES OF RESEARCH IN NURSING

Research in nursing serves several purposes, all of which at different times may have particular relevance to the Clinical Nurse Specialist. The main ones are discussed below.

To establish scientifically defensible reasons for nursing activities

Clinical Nurse Specialists are at the forefront of developments in their speciality and so must be prepared to argue for the introduction of research-based developments with both nursing colleagues, doctors and other health-care professionals. To do this effectively they must be confident of the soundness of the research and its relevance to their area of practice.

To find ways of increasing the cost effectiveness of nursing activities

As Henderson and Nite (1978) stated

> "Nursing ... born in the church and bred in the military, has relied heavily on authority and tradition, not to mention intuition ... and most aspects of nursing are steeped in tradition and passed on, unchanged and unchanging from one generation to another – too often they are routine and without rhyme or reason."

Unfortunately much nursing practice is still not cost effective. Activities are undertaken in a ritualistic fashion which are wasteful of the nurses' time, for example, the routine recording of temperature, pulse, respirations and blood pressure unnecessarily or with equipment which does not work properly, despite research evidence to demonstrate the limitations of such activity. In addition, critical research findings related to control of the spread of infection such as hand washing and the cleaning of patients' washbowls are ignored, which may mean nurses are wasting time on activities which are not effective. Clinical Nurse Specialists are in an ideal position to influence clinical practice in all the areas they work by encouraging a research base for nursing practice, making it more cost effective.

To satisfy the academic curiosity of thinking nurses

Although all would agree that this should be a prime reason for undertaking research it is the least common in nursing. One reason for this is the lack of funding for research which does not have some practical outcome for those supporting it. Academic curiosity is probably the foundation of all nursing research but the need for funding means this reason does not appear on applications for funding as it could be interpreted as selfish rather than for the benefit of patient care.

To provide evidence of weakness and strength in nursing

One of the anxieties which nurses who are the subject of research have is that their practice will be found to be inadequate in some respect. Certainly this is sometimes the case, but what should be borne in mind is that the purpose of much nursing research, as stated above, is about improving the quality of care that patients receive, which should include being willing to recognise defects in current nursing practice. Having said that, nursing research does also highlight areas of good practice which should include being willing to recognise deficits in current nursing practice, and which can then act as examples for others.

To provide evidence in support of demands for resources in nursing

This is particularly pertinent in the current funding policies in the National Health Service. Resources include people, equipment and procedures. The NHS is the largest single employer in Europe and about 50% of the National Health Service budget is spent on staffing, which makes it essential that the best possible skill mix is achieved. This entails ensuring that the right people, those with the necessary skills for the task, are in the right place at the right time. The difficulty is that identifying skills, and quantifying them, is not easy and so many reports have avoided the issue by discussing grades rather than skills. However,

Clinical Nurse Specialists are skilled practitioners and it is important that they can demonstrate the benefit of their contribution to the quality of patient care, and the possible additional costs if their services are withdrawn. For example, when patients develop complications which will be expensive to treat, such as diabetes, rheumatoid arthritis or a stoma, the difference could be demonstrated by comparing patient outcomes in those units or districts/trusts where a Clinical Nurse Specialist is employed with those where there is no Clinical Nurse Specialist for a particular speciality. Equipment may also be an expensive purchase and again the argument must be about the balance between the initial cost of equipment and its maintenance, compared with the cost especially in terms of patient welfare, but also of additional demands that may be placed on ward or community staff if the equipment is not provided. Finally hospital and community procedures may be restrictive and do not allow the Clinical Nurse Specialist to function as an independent practitioner, which is a waste of such a valuable resource. Therefore it is important that the Clinical Nurse Specialist can argue for the right to exercise professional autonomy, and part of the argument must come from study of available research evidence.

To earn and defend a professional status for nursing

In 1973 Catherine Hall, of the Royal College of Nursing identified what she believed were the main characteristics of a profession. These included that a profession:

- provides a service to society, involving specialised knowledge and skills;
- possesses a unique body of knowledge;
- sets its own standards;
- adapts its services to meet changing needs;
- accepts responsibility for safeguarding the clients it serves;
- strives to make economical use of its·practitioners.

All of this has particular relevance for the Clinical Nurse Specialist who provides a specialist service, and whose practice must be research based. The Clinical Nurse Specialist may choose to undertake research to improve practice, become an informed consumer of research, disseminate research findings to colleagues, or encourage others to undertake research. To achieve any of these requires at least an understanding of the research process and an ability to read a research report critically.

THE RESEARCH PROCESS

The conduct of research will vary depending upon the subject, purpose and subject(s) of the research; such research must be a systematic, scientific process, (Clark and Hockey, 1979) therefore the whole project must be carefully planned. Abdellah and Levine (1986) identify 12 major steps in the research process, though they emphasise that not every project requires consideration of all the steps. Listed in order of logical development of a project these steps are:

1. Select the topic and formulate the problem
2. Review the literature
3. Formulate a framework of theory
4. Formulate hypotheses
5. Define the variables and determine how they will be quantified
6. Develop the research design
7. Define the study population and sample
8. Determine how to collect the data
9. Determine how to process and summarise the data
10. Formulate the data analysis
11. Formulate interpretation of data
12. Determine the method of communicating the results.

1. Select the topic and formulate the problem

First, of course, comes the idea. An essential virtue for a successful researcher is the 'satiable curiosity' of Kipling's Elephant's Child who said:

"I keep six honest serving-men
(They taught me all I knew)
Their names are What and Why and When
And How and Where and Who"

After selecting the topic for study this should then be refined to turn it into a manageable problem. For example, whether working in hospital or the community, a topic of interest may be preparation for discharge and its impact on the patient's/client's future progress; or when caring for someone who is dying, the concern may be if it is better or not to tell a patient that they are terminally ill.

2. Review the literature

Next it is necessary to find out what other research has been undertaken in your selected area of study; however, be warned, a well conducted literature search is very time consuming, and often frustrating. First it must be established whether or not the study being contemplated has already been undertaken. If this is the case then there are two options available: either to adopt the results of the research, assuming it is sound (see a later section which deals with critically reading research reports), or to replicate the study to confirm the findings and their relevance to a specific area of practice.

3. Formulate a framework of theory

A theory is a set of sentences whose purpose is to explain (Roy and Roberts, 1981), and in research terms a theory must be proved to be correct, but it must also be recognised that theories are subject to change. Therefore one of the functions of research is to revise or reformulate existing theory, which often has not provided satisfactory explanation of phenomena, by producing new knowledge (Abdellah and Levine, 1986), and this can be a key area of research for the Clinical Nurse Specialist.

4. Formulate hypotheses

A hypothesis is 'a statement of the expected relationship(s) among the phenomena being studied' (Abdellah and Levine, 1986). For example between information giving and patient care outcomes (Boore, 1978; Hayward, 1981), or patient participation in goal setting and improved care outcomes (Horsley *et al.*, 1981). Crow (1980) wanted to see if there was a difference in performance between the Bachelor of Nursing student and the Pre-registration Nursing student in identifying nursing problems and suggesting nursing interventions. One of her hypotheses was that:

"The ability of nurses to suggest nursing interventions for identified problems depends on:
a) their training scheme;
b) their utilisation of convergent or divergent thinking styles;
c) whether their teachers encourage creative personalities."

Crow (1980) used a variety of tests in her study, but not all nursing research questions are amenable to an experimental research approach. An alternative to experimentation, which is more appropriate for studying nurses and nursing, is action research, where a phenomenen is studied, changes introduced and the results of those changes studied (hopefully to demonstrate an improvement). For example, Metcalf

(1983) studied the effects of the change in the delivery of nursing care in the ward of a maternity hospital from task allocation to patient-centred care. This type of study is one which newly appointed Clinical Nurse Specialists could use to demonstrate the impact their appointment has had on the quality of patient care.

However, there is also a need for descriptive or explanatory studies, styles of research which at one time were considered to be weak compared with the rigours of the experimental, scientific approach, but are gradually being recognised as worthy and necessary. Gallego (1983) argued forcibly for the value and benefit of descriptive, qualitative research. According to Brink and Wood (1988) the basic difference is that 'what' questions invariably lead to descriptive designs: 'why' questions are always experimental. Brykczyńska (1987) reviewed therapeutic and non-therapeutic research with children and the ethical and legal implications for nurses and nurse researchers, and Crow and Clark (1987) studied the development of standards through implementing research which would make a contribution to quality assurance. The first study could be replicated by a Clinical Nurse Specialist working in other clinical settings, which is acceptable as long as appropriate permission is granted, and the results of the latter study apply in any clinical setting and therefore could be beneficial to Clinical Nurse Specialists in several aspects of their work.

5. Define the variables and determine how they will be quantified

The definition of variables (phenomena being studied) has to be completed before any data are collected but only apply in experimental investigations for properties that are being studied and which can vary, such as age, sex, height, performance and activities. As Partridge and Barnitt (1986) explain, some variables such as sex are mutually exclusive, for example if you are male you cannot also be female (except in rarest circumstances). Other variables, such as height or weight, can be measured along a continuum. The independent variable refers to the variables that are being manipulated, and a study examines the effect of manipulating these on the dependent variable. An example is the relationship between self-esteem, perceived health status, age, sex, education, income and health-promotive lifestyle in older, non-institutionalised persons (Hanner, 1987). At this stage if the data require statistical analysis it is essential that a statistician is consulted, for their advice could positively influence the research design and save a lot of grief later.

6. Develop the research design

The research design depends on whether the study is experimental, historical/retrospective or survey, the style adopted determines the best way to answer the questions the researcher is asking.

Experiment

Briefly, (a) an experimental study requires that two groups of subjects are selected who are matched for all those characteristics which are relevant to the study. For example, initially Boore's subjects (Boore, 1978) were paired on the basis of three criteria: sex, operation and consultant under whose care the patient was admitted. (b) One group, the experimental group, is exposed to a treatment, the other acts as the control group; Boore's experimental group received information about its operation in a planned interview lasting about 35 minutes, and was taught simple post-operative exercises. The control group was visited and the patient and researcher talked about topics unrelated to hospital for about the same period of time. (c) The pre-determined outcomes for the two groups are compared. Boore used three objective measurements: temperature, analgesic consumption and incidence of complications; one biochemical indicator: the excretion of 17-hydroxycorticosteroids; and three subjective scales: assessment of mental and physical state, pain and medical and nursing assessments. She then compared the results of the measurements between the experimental and control groups.

Historical or retrospective

Both these research styles are concerned with events which occurred in the past. Historical studies use either people's recollections of events, or make use of written records. Such work was undertaken by Monica Baly (1977) and Joyce Prince (1984). The historical researcher seeks to establish truth, ascertain facts and form the basis of conclusions and generalisations. As they both demonstrated, what is all important is that historiographers compare documents with the originals and whenever possible use primary sources (Abdellah and Levine, 1986). This style of research may be of interest to the Clinical Nurse Specialist who wishes to examine the development of the Clinical Nurse Specialist role. Retrospective studies are used by epidemiologists to describe a study in which the effect is known, for example lung cancer, and the cause is sought. This is achieved by checking statistics relating to incidence of the 'effect' and seeking causal relationships, such as between lung

37

cancer and smoking, or the spread of HIV/AIDS and unprotected sexual intercourse, drug addicts sharing needles, or transfusion with contaminated blood or blood products. Again this style of research may be useful to the Clinical Nurse Specialist either to further explore the area of clinical specialism, or to study the impact of the introduction of the Clinical Nurse Specialist within a particular health care setting.

Survey

This is a design for research in which the purpose is to gather information about a large number of people by collecting data from a few (Holm and Llewellyn, 1986), the principal methods of data collection being interviews, observation, questionnaires or any combination of the three. However, according to Holm and Llewellyn (1986)

> "Regardless of specific objectives, a survey should meet certain standards or indicators of quality. One of these is related to sampling. Because a survey aims to describe a population based on information from a select few, it is essential that the sample obtained is representative of the population."

Thus, if the study is of all qualified nurses caring for the elderly in designated units in general hospitals (the population), then nurses working in the community or in psychiatric hospitals cannot be included as they are not representative of the population.

7. Define the study population and sample

> "The first step of the sampling process is the identification of the population from which the sample will be drawn. The *population* is the entire set of individuals or elements defined by the sampling criteria established for the study. The sample is then chosen from the study population."

(Burns and Grove, 1987)

Thus the findings can then be generalised to the population as a whole. Generalising means that the findings are expected to describe not only the sample but also the target population from which the sample was taken. So that if for example the Clinical Nurse Specialist's specialism is rheumatology and the purpose is to study some aspect of the impact of Clinical Nurse Specialists' interventions on patient care, then quite obviously patients with other disorders cannot be included in the study. However, if the area of interest is more general and aims to include any patients/clients who are cared for, or whose care is directed, by a Clinical Nurse Specialist, whatever the specialism, then the sample must be representative of this population for such variables as age, sex and incidence of specialism within the total population.

8. Determine how to collect the data

Types of data to be collected can be generalised according to whether they are collected as qualitative – research with a systematic, subjective approach used to describe life experiences and give them meaning, or quantitative – a formal, objective, systematic process for obtaining information about the world. This research method is used to describe, test relationships, and examine cause and effect relationships (Brink and Wood, 1988). In the past much nursing research, because of the phenomena being studied, has been qualitative and as such has been criticised as being weak and 'unscientific', however, the benefit of this approach to research design in the health care setting is gaining acceptance and credibility. As stated above, data collection may be through the use of secondary data, observation, interviews or questionnaires, or any combination of these. However, important features which must be taken into account when determining how to collect the data are halo effect, stereotyping, Hawthorne effect and bias.

"Halo effect may occur when the interviewer allows their perception of one characteristic of the interviewee ... to influence their interpretation of other aspects, the first impression often having the strongest effect."
(Partridge and Barnitt, 1986)

Akin to this is stereotyping which may occur when the interviewer forms a faulty impression of the interviewee because of their clothes, accent or mannerisms. The Hawthorne effect is a phenomenon whereby changes will occur in the performance of data subjects primarily because they are participating in the study and not as a result of the factors being studied. For example, patients/clients health care outcomes may improve because of the increased interest in them and their well-being rather than because a new treatment has been introduced which is being monitored. Bias can be introduced into a study at any point from the initial writing of the research question to the final conclusions of the research report. This should be guarded against and it is for this reason that critical comment should be sought from an independent observer at all stages.

9. Determine how to process and summarise the data

As stated earlier it is essential that the advice of a statistician is sought at the first stage of the research process and that the statistician is consulted at each successive stage. Quantitative research by definition requires rigorous statistical analysis, using parametric tests, and the statistician should advise on the research design which will produce the strongest test results. However, qualitative research may also be susceptible to statistical analysis. It will depend on the volume of data generated, and the complexity of the statistical analysis to be undertaken, whether computer facilities will need to be used. As an aside, whatever method of data analysis is selected – computer or manual – it is expensive and time-consuming and this should be taken into account when costing the project.

10, 11. Determine how to process, summarise and interpret data

Data analysis is part of the interpretive phase of the research process and consists of arranging all the information so that it tells something about the research question. Data analysis is: categorising, ordering, manipulating and summarising the data in order to obtain answers to the research question (Kerlinger, 1973). However, Abdellah and Levine (1986) stress that: "It is essential that the method by which the data are to be processed be decided in advance of data collection ... (and) summarising data consists of converting raw data into an orderly and 'digestible' body of knowledge." The summary may include producing tables, diagrams, graphs and the allocation of issues and ideas into selected categories. Interpretation consists of examining the evidence, considering the implications, exploring the significance of the findings, and generalising findings in respect of the original research question, thus drawing meaning from data (Abdellah and Levine, 1986).

12. Determine the method of communicating the results

This final stage of the research process is often neglected, and yet it is the most important as, without dissemination, research findings cannot be critiqued and then utilised. A well written research report should include:

- a statement regarding the purpose of the study;
- a review of the literature;
- information about sampling;
- a description of the data collection method;
- a description of statistical analysis;
- a description of pilot studies;

- copies of questionnaires/interview schedules;
- findings from which conclusions are derived.

The actual research should be reported in sufficient detail that the study can be replicated, that is, reproduced in the same form as the original work to confirm the findings. In this way, the results cannot be falsified, and if a mistake has been made or information regarding the conduct of the research is missing, it will not be possible to reproduce the study due to this lack of information. A variety of methods of presentation should be used as it is important to communicate findings to the widest possible audience, including nurse researchers, nurse practitioners, nurse educators, nurse managers and students of nursing, as well as other health care professionals.

Communication of findings should include publication in a range of nursing journals and the style of the publication should be modified to suit the intended audience. If, for example, the research was undertaken for the award of a higher degree then a copy of the original dissertation should be lodged in the Steinberg Collection in the Royal College of Nursing Library. Reports should be submitted for publication in journals which have a special interest in research, such as *Nursing Research* or the *Journal of Advanced Nursing*. In addition, reports should be published in appropriate specialist journals, and in the more popular nursing journals. The style of presentation should, of course, be suitable for the selected audience, and all journals provide guidelines on house style and content. Articles submitted for publication are vetted by critical readers, which is most helpful to the novice author.

In addition, oral and visual presentation at conferences, study days, workshops and seminars is necessary to audiences who are interested in the research process itself and to audiences who are interested in the specialist subject matter of the research. The advantage of attending the former events is that it provides an opportunity to share experiences with other researchers which can be invaluable; peer group support is also available through membership of a local nursing research interest group or the Royal College of Nursing Research Advisory Group. Information about such events, be they research or specialist, local, national or international, is published in many nursing journals and the call for abstracts is published well in advance of the event. Communicating research findings and sharing the experience is essential for the professional development of nursing and for the improvement in the quality of patient care. Holm and Llewellyn (1986) identify seven ways of communicating information about research which could be undertaken either by the researcher or by a Clinical Nurse Specialist interested in promoting the utilisation of research findings:

1. Volunteer to conduct an in-service training programme
2. Write an article for publication
3. Use creative approaches to problem identification
4. Increase contact with other health care professionals outside nursing
5. Become an active member of a professional organisation such as the Royal College of Nursing Research Advisory Group
6. Participate in workshops, conferences and conventions
7. Read professional journals.

ETHICS AND NURSING RESEARCH

To some extent the United Kingdom Central Council's (UKCC) Code of Professional Conduct establishes the standards for nurses involved in nursing research. This involvement may occur at three levels: (1) nurses undertaking research; (2) nurses in a position of responsibility where research is being carried out; (3) nurses practising in places where research is being carried out (Royal College of Nursing, 1993). Cormack (1984) summarises the first section as follows:

1. The research must be necessary and must contribute to further knowledge.
2. The subjects must receive full explanations of what their participation might entail and must be told explicitly that they have the right to refuse.
3. Consent must be obtained, if necessary, from a relative or legal guardian.
4. Subjects must be protected against physical, emotional, mental or social injury; confidentiality must be assured and maintained.
5. The researcher must be qualified to carry out the investigation, and must make public the results of the inquiry and must attempt to prevent their misuse.
6. The contract between the sponsor of the research and the researcher must make explicit their mutual obligations and must state clearly the remit for the work to be undertaken.
7. Clear arrangements must be made as to the researcher's duties and responsibilities in the place where the research is carried out.

However, it should be borne in mind that

"it can often be difficult for a patient to refuse to participate in anything proposed by those responsible for their care treatment. Acquiescence must never be taken for granted."

(Partridge and Barnitt, 1986).

The second part of the Royal College of Nursing guidelines provides advice on sanctioning or commissioning research, and emphasises that consent to participate cannot be given on behalf of other people. The third part reminds nurses of their responsibilities as practitioners to safeguard patients'/clients' rights and well-being, as it emphasises the fact that nurses who agree to assist with data collection are bound by the same obligations as the researcher (Cormack, 1984). Where research involves accessing patient records then permission must be obtained from "the doctor or other clinician who made the records and from the medical records department" (Partridge and Barnitt, 1986). In its *Issues in Nursing and Health* series published by the Royal College of Nursing, No. 2 deals with the issue of 'Patient records and research – a position statement' and No. 3 with 'Research trials – advice for nurses and nursing students', both of which are recommended reading (Royal College of Nursing, 1992). In addition, data extracted and processed must meet the requirements of the *Data Protection Act 1984*.

Finally, a proposal for any research involving people (human subjects) must be submitted to the relevant Local Research Ethics Committee. The function of these committees is to consider the ethics of proposed research projects which will involve human subjects, and which will take place broadly within the National Health Service. The Local Research Ethics Committee's task is to advise the National Health Service body under whose auspices the research is intended to take place (Department of Health, 1991). However, Julia Neuberger (1992) pursues the issue of the role of ethics committees further, and for those Clinical Nurse Specialists involved in research in any capacity her report should be essential reading.

CRITIQUING A RESEARCH REPORT

In order to critique a research report the Clinical Nurse Specialist must be familiar with the research process. Chapman (in Cormack, 1984) suggests that the evaluation should be:

1. *Objective*. The person carrying out the critique must not criticise just because they do not like the findings, nor because they go against common beliefs or attitudes. The criticism must be based on factual material and be supported by facts. It is important to criticise the research and not the researcher.
2. *Constructive*. Criticism can easily be destructive when only negative things are commented upon and no credit is given for any good points; strengths as well as weakness should be revealed. It is also

possible to show that while a particular piece of work may not be acceptable as it stands, small adjustments either in presentation or approach may make it of greater value.

3. *Penetrating.* Superficially a piece of work may appear valuable and only when examined more deeply may flaws be revealed. The evaluation must be honest in that the person carrying it out must be prepared to state clearly why a point is good or bad. It is not honest to fall back on such phrases as 'it appears'; opinions must be supported by facts.

4. *Value free.* Bias is almost certain to be present in the person undertaking the critique, in the same way as it may be present in the researcher. This means that any strongly held attitudes should be acknowledged so that the bias is recognised.

5. *Decisive.* When the work has been read in this manner, it is important to summarise the appraisal and to assess whether any flaws are substantive or are only minor issues. A decision has to be made as to whether, despite defects, the findings are acceptable.

CONCLUSION

It has long been recognised that in the pursuit of professional status nursing must become research based, and the Clinical Nurse Specialist should be the vanguard, setting an example for colleagues. The Clinical Nurse Specialist should be involved in research and encourage colleagues to utilise research findings, because it is clinically desirable, so that patients should receive the highest standard of care available. Hence it is professionally, and ethically, desirable so that care givers meet the standards of the *United Kingdom Central Council Code of Professional Conduct* (1992), and defensible in law, to ensure that no case of negligence could be brought because care given to a patient was not based on research findings. A classic example would be the case of a patient who developed pressure sores while in hospital and subsequently sued the ward sister for negligence. Pressure sore prevention and treatment is one of the most extensively researched areas of nursing care, one of the earliest studies being the work of Norton *et al.* (1962), and yet pressure sores are still accepted by some nurses as inevitable in certain cases.

For the Clinical Nurse Specialist to encourage the utilisation of research findings requires an understanding of the change process. Stages in the process of planned change, based on Lippitt (1972) are:

1. Determining the need for change by comparing the desired state with the current state in the delivery or outcome of nursing care.

2. Assessment of the motivation and commitment of all those involved to the proposed change.
3. Assessment of the resources required to facilitate the proposed change including equipment, communication networks, manpower and teaching.
4. Setting objectives for change, which should be realistic and achievable, which may mean that the change should be introduced in stages.
5. Establishing the roles of facilitators and those participating in change, leaders, teachers, and those implementing the proposed change.
6. Maintaining change once initiated. Only if staff have accepted the need for change, understood its purpose and appreciate the benefit to patients will innovation become part of the culture.
7. Withdrawal of the facilitator, at which time the staff should be able to continue the change on its own initiative and the facilitator is willing to allow this freedom and 'let go'.

Both the conduct and utilisation of research are a challenge to the Clinical Nurse Specialist. However, as Hockey (1979) exhorted:

"A serious commitment to research has serious implications which need to be faced and which affect every member of the profession. The most important implication must be a willingness to appraise research findings seriously and to use them as and when appropriate ... Professional practice must be defensible professionally, ethically and legally."

And this is the enduring challenge for Clinical Nurse Specialists who are at the forefront of nursing in their specialism.

REFERENCES

Abdellah F.G. and Levine E. (1986) *Better Patient Care Through Nursing Research*. Macmillan, London.
Baly M. (1977) *Nursing*. Batsford, London.
Boore J.P.R. (1978) *Prescription for Recovery*. Royal College of Nursing, London.
Briggs Report (1972) *Report of the Committee on Nursing*. HMSO, London.
Brink P.J. and Wood M.J. (1988) *Basic Steps in Planning Nursing Research*. Jones and Bartlett, Boston, Massachusetts.
Brykczyńska M-M. (1987) In *Clinical Excellence in Nursing – International Networking* (Conference Abstracts). Royal College of Nursing, London.
Burnard P. and Chapman C.M. (1990) *Nurse Education: The Way Forward*. Scutari, London.
Burns N. and Grove S.K. (1987) *The Practice of Nursing Research*. Saunders, Philadelphia, Pennsylvania.

Clark J.M. and Hockey L. (1979) *Research for Nursing*. HM+M Publishers, Aylesbury.

Cormack D. (1984) *The Research Process in Nursing*. Blackwell Scientific, Oxford.

Crow J. (1980) *Effects of Preparation on Problem Solving*. Royal College of Nursing, London.

Crow M. and Clark M. (1987) Developing standards through implementing research: a contribution to quality assurance. In Brykczyńska M-M. (1987).

Department of Health (1991) *Local Ethics Committees* 8 HS9(91) 5 Aug. HMSO, London.

Gallego A.P. (1983) *Evaluating the School, A Case Study in the Evaluation of a School of Nursing*. Royal College of Nursing, London.

Hanner M.B. (1987) Factors related to promotion of health: seeking behaviours in the aged. In Brykczyńska M-M. (1987).

Hayward J. (1981) *Information – A Prescription Against Pain*. Royal College of Nursing, London.

Henderson V. and Nite G. (1978) *Principles and Practice of Nursing*. Macmillan, London.

Hockey L. (1979) Expanding the nursing horizons. *Nursing Mirror*, October 25.

Holm K. and Llewellyn J.G. (1986) *Nursing Research for Nursing Practice*. Saunders, Philadelphia, Pennsylvania.

Horsley J.A. *et al.* (1981) *Using Research to Improve Nursing Practice*. Grune and Stratton, London.

Kerlinger F.N. (1973) In Castles M.R. (Ed.), *Primer of Nursing Research*. Saunders, Philadelphia, Pennsylvania.

Lippitt (1972) cited in Farmer E.S. (1983) Planned change in nursing. Occasional Paper 29(9). *Nursing Times*, 79(16): 41–44.

Metcalf C. (1983) In *Nursing Research – Ten Studies in Nursing Care*. Wiley, Chichester.

Neuberger J. (1992) *Ethics and Health Care – The Role of Research Ethics Committees in the United Kingdom*. King's Fund Institute, London.

Norton D. *et al.* (1962) *An Investigation of Geriatric Nursing Problems in Hospital*. Churchill Livingstone, Edinburgh (1975). Originally published 1962 by National Corporation for the Care of Old People, London.

Partridge C.J. and Barnitt R.E. (1986) *Research Guidelines: A Handbook for Therapists*. Heinemann Physiotherapy, London.

Prince J. (1984) *Miss Nightingale's Vision of a Nursing Profession*. 3rd Annual Winifred Raphael Memorial Lecture. Royal College of Nursing, London.

Roy C. and Roberts S.L. (1981) *Theory Construction in Nursing*. Prentice-Hall, Englewood Cliffs, New Jersey.

Royal College of Nursing (1992) *Issues in Nursing and Health, No. 2* and *No. 3*. RCN, London.

Royal College of Nursing (1993) *Ethics Related to Research in Nursing*. RCN, London.

CHAPTER FOUR

Educator: telling or selling?

Debra Humphris and Caroline Soar

Probably the most influential role of the Clinical Nurse Specialist is that of educator, for it is an element which consumes a considerable amount of the role, involving clients, carers and colleagues. The purpose of the interaction of Clinical Nurse Specialists as educators with their client group is to enable individuals to sustain their optimal lifestyle through a process of empowerment. However, is the locus of the educator role entirely about empowering and enabling individuals to maintain or regain integrity and self-care? Or is the expectation also to ensure and promote individual compliance with therapeutic regimes through the strategies of both telling and selling? A major assumption underpinning the educator role is the desire for individuals to comply with appropriate therapeutic regimes. If this is the purpose of education then there is a fine line between enabling and ensuring. If education is about empowering people, then to what extent do individuals have the opportunity to question and influence changes in their therapeutic regime? Education should encourage questioning and curiosity within individuals, however there may be times when training is the most appropriate strategy. Indeed, if the process of education is to foster a more questioning approach, is the health care organisation prepared to deal with the issues that arise? As education is a life-long process, then there must be constant adaptation and responsiveness in order to deliver a contemporary service. Consequently, the Clinical Nurse Specialist has a professional obligation constantly to update skills and knowledge, resulting in resource implications which must be considered.

This chapter does not set out to deal with the *how* to educate or teach, as these issues are dealt with extensively elsewhere in the literature. The intention is to explore some of the issues related to the educator role of the Clinical Nurse Specialist. In doing so, particular dilemmas will be discussed to illustrate the power that the Clinical Nurse Specialist exercises through this role. The intention is to question a number of assumptions, as well as asking how effective is educational activity?

WHAT IS EDUCATION – COMPETENCE OR COMPLIANCE?

A fundamental question the Clinical Nurse Specialist must consider in relation to the role of educator is: should the Clinical Nurse Specialist educate or train other people? Perhaps before attempting to answer this question, it may be helpful to define what is meant by 'education' in order to give meaning, and thus direct the line of enquiry.

There are many definitions of education depending on an individual's beliefs in either the classical or romantic model of education. Nursing philosophy in the 1990s is focused on a holistic approach to care, and part of the holistic approach is dependent on a humanistic element being present. This element is usually written as part of a clinical area's philosophy. Humanism is about accepting individuals as having dignity and worth, capable of making choices. It is more concerned with the individual rather than social morals, and the emphasis is on the person's drive for growth and development, as well as having some control over personal destiny. Therefore, education would best be defined in humanistic terms. Jarvis (1983) suggests that "education is any planned series of incidents, having a humanistic basis, directed towards the participant(s) learning and understanding." To explore this definition further, it is obvious that fundamental to education is the presence of understanding. Understanding is more important than learning, as it is concerned with the conceptualising and internalising of knowledge. Learning is bringing about a change in behaviour which does not necessarily demand understanding. For example, the Clinical Nurse Specialist may teach a patient a particular task such as the administration of a certain medication at a certain time. The individual learns how to do this, but if the reason *why* is not made clear, learning has occurred but not understanding. There has been a considerable amount of debate about the notion of should we educate or should we train. To train someone is to teach them to do something without necessarily understanding why. To return to the question posed earlier, it would seem rather incongruous and perhaps unethical to train individuals, if philosophies and value statements lend themselves towards a holistic approach to care being in essence humanistic. If one role of the Clinical Nurse Specialist is to empower the individual, which will be discussed further on in the text, then the Clinical Nurse Specialist's role is to educate, not to train.

Another question that should now be considered is: what is the Clinical Nurse Specialist educating people for? Again before considering the question, it is necessary to identify who the recipients of education are. The two broad groups are the givers of care and the receivers of care. The givers of care include health care professional, relatives, partners and anyone involved in the individual's care. The receivers of care are the individuals themselves, but may also include relatives and partners. There may be a need to educate to differing levels depending on need, prior knowledge and perceived ability to understand. However, the approaches to individuals in whichever group should be consistent with the values of the educational process adopted. The Clinical Nurse Specialist should consider that neither group is hierarchical, nor does one group deserve more in-depth knowledge than the other, because depth of knowledge is a subjective matter and will depend on the level of understanding the recipient of education has.

One of the functions of education is to enable the participant to reach a level of competence. Competence is quite simply having a level, or a standard of ability, and in order to reach this, it is necessary to have the required skill and knowledge to prove competence; a prerequisite for any issues concerning education is the presence of consent. The factors for the Clinical Nurse Specialist to consider in this are twofold. The first is consent to undertake the education on offer, which concerns the recipient understanding what is involved and the consequences, both personal and otherwise, arising from this. This first stage is usually concerned with the imparting of knowledge and information. For example, in a clinical scenario, the Clinical Nurse Specialist may impart knowledge and information about a certain proposed method of treatment. The recipient in this case will, after having received this education, understand the process and consequences of treatment. Education may then become involved in the context of the second stage of consent.

In the second stage, the recipient receives what might be termed an ethical education. This concerns the conveyance of not only information but also of the rights the recipient has to make decisions and choices about what to do with the information conveyed in the first stage. To draw further on the earlier example, the individuals, having received information about the process and consequences of treatment, are now educated to a level whereby they understand the range of rights and options relevant to their current scenario. This does not necessarily mean that they are empowered, since the information may have been conveyed in a manner which deters them from exercising those rights.

This may be the professional's way of ensuring patient compliance. Dracup and Meleis (1982) defined compliance as "the extent to which

49

an individual chooses behaviours that coincide with a clinical prescription," and they further suggest that compliance is enhanced if the compliant role is reinforced by significant others and other reference groups. If the person chooses behaviours that do not coincide with the clinical prescription, two effects may occur. Firstly the clinical prescription becomes meaningless, and perhaps as a direct result of this, negative labels are given to the non-compliant person.

Negative labelling tends to have the effect of avoidance of the individual by the professionals, who may adopt defensive behaviour, and employ paternalistic caring strategies. The professionals tend to listen less, or listen selectively to what they wish to hear. The professionals may tend to over-compensate with other individuals requiring their services to prove their worth, and continually to justify their role. There may also exist a lack of trust and honesty between the professionals and the individuals.

The Clinical Nurse Specialist needs to understand that the notion of non-compliance is a very real side-effect of the educational process. Consequently if the Clinical Nurse Specialist is truly to act as an educator, the convincing imparting of information is not enough to complete the education process. In order for that information to have meaningful impact on the recipient, that individual must be able to feel and demonstrate empowerment.

EMPOWERMENT AND PATERNALISM

A central element of the educator role of the Clinical Nurse Specialist is the empowering of individuals, which is the process by which people are able to experience and exercise autonomy. Empowerment has been defined as "to authorise or enable" (*Oxford English Dictionary*). The increasing emphasis placed on the concepts of partnership and self-care can be witnessed by the commonplace use of such language in nursing, for as Ashworth *et al.* (1992) argue, there is a need for a fundamental clarification of the 'nature of participation'.

Many people requiring the interventions of a Clinical Nurse Specialist develop a knowledge-base about coping with their own needs. Their own repertoire of strategies may well be superior to those provided by many health care professionals. However, the Clinical Nurse Specialist is in a position to assist the individual constantly to enhance and develop new self-caring behaviours. The concept of self-care as set out by Orem (1991) suggested that self-care is a series of learned behaviours, to which the individual constantly adds as a result of a range of internal and external factors. The exercise of self-care requires, as Orem (1991) states, "both learning and the use of knowledge as well as enduring motivation and skill;" and it is by this process individuals enable themselves and others. One assumption underpinning any process of empowerment is that every individual, when confronted with a situation of health deviation, actually wishes to, or is able to become empowered.

Waterworth and Luker (1990) in exploring the concept of collaboration in care suggested that people "may not wish to become involved in decisions about their care." While acknowledging that there is evidence to suggest that people's active involvement in their own care may improve outcomes (Wilson-Barnett and Fordham, 1982), they too, went on to suggest that even if people are well informed, they may not want to be involved in making decisions about their care. From their research they identified the notion of 'toeing the line', where people were concerned to do the right thing, one consequence of this willingness being that

"staff may, if they adopt practices which encourage involvement, unwittingly coerce patients to comply."

(Waterworth and Luker, 1990)

Therefore, the assumption that all members of the population are willing to, or desire to be empowered and involved in decision making about their care, clearly needs to be explored. Indeed, Altschul (1983) suggested that individuals may require help both in "exercising their right to learn or not to learn." Clinical Nurse Specialists can exercise considerable influence over this process, both by helping to meet the needs of each individual through acting as an agent of optimal self-care, as well as by acting to give authority. This could be achieved by negotiating and defining reasonable limits of action, while avoiding the creation of unrealistic expectations of individual health status. A consequence of such empowerment must be the engagement of the Clinical Nurse Specialist in the debate about the provision and availability of services. Historically, the perception of the individual as a passive and grateful recipient of all interventions is shifting from a paternalistic mode to that of empowerment, with individuals actively engaged in the process of their care. While this may be viewed as a desirable state of affairs, Waterworth and Luker (1990) offer a salient reminder that such a shift of responsibility clearly has economic implications for both the individual and the Health Service. Indeed it is appropriate to recall that this shift is only for those people using the health services, given that "most illnesses are treated by self-care or by informal care provided by relatives and friends" (Pollitt, 1984).

WHO HOLDS CONTROL?

The process of empowerment through education raises questions about the balance of control in the interactions between the individual and the health care system. As therapeutic regimes become increasingly complex, so the individual requires a greater degree and amount of information (Oberst, 1989). Associated with this are the issues of motivation and the individual's belief that what happens to them can be influenced by their own behaviour. Antonovsky (1992) characterises this as 'integrity', and in so doing, exposes the assumption of the importance placed on the individual's willingness, and ability, to exercise responsibility and initiative in self-care. A readiness to learn and motivation, Davidhizar (1983) suggests, are influenced by an awareness of one's susceptibility to disease, with a strong negative perception acting as a barrier to action. Without the individuals' motivation and belief in their ability to exercise control, the process of education is unlikely to be successful (Wilson-Barnett and Batehup, 1988). The individuals' perception of the severity or threat of their disorder can be significantly influenced by the Clinical Nurse Specialist, with differing perceptions resulting in altered levels of motivation. Therefore, the Clinical Nurse Specialist has to manage this fine balance between the positive and negative aspects of each individual's disorder, constantly maintaining a sense of realism. The educator role needs to remain focused on enabling individuals to merge the necessary health care behaviours into their everyday life (Smith, 1989).

Breaking the news about an individual's diagnosis remains the responsibility of medical practitioners. However, the interdependent nature of the Doctor/Clinical Nurse Specialist relationship may place Clinical Nurse Specialists in a precarious position, as they attempt to maintain the delicate balance between withholding information and exceeding the responsibilities of the role. This leads to the question of whether it is really feasible that control can move into the individual's hands through the process of education, or is it a tacit desire to maximise compliance (Waterworth and Luker, 1990)? A constant dilemma faced by the Clinical Nurse Specialist is to what extent the educator role is: to what extent is the educator role about training to enhance compliance with medically prescribed regimes, or is it a genuine process of empowerment and democratisation of health care? As the interventions delivered within this role shift between these two extremes, the Clinical Nurse Specialist has constantly to strike a balance, for each individual, between telling and selling a package of care.

Clinical Nurse Specialists are in a pivotal position to make judgements about whether or not individuals are competent in dealing with their health care needs. Anderson and Elfert (1989), in their study of chronically ill children, suggest that the consequences of the mother not displaying competence in caring for the child, and thus being labelled an 'unfit mother', were far-reaching for both the family and the child. This places pressures on the carer to meet societal expectations, for failing to do so may result in the intervention of the state authorities. In Western society the possession of knowledge, Fleming (1992) argues, places individuals in a "higher position", resulting in the creation of interdependence of those who do not possess the knowledge. Fleming (1992) goes on to suggest that this situation is viewed by many "as the natural order of things" and as such they are unwilling to contradict the situation, clearly echoing Waterworth and Luker's (1990) notion of "toeing the line". If the Clinical Nurse Specialist is to make an effective impact as an educator of people, there is a need to promote a greater dialogue about the very nature of the Clinical Nurse Specialist–client relationship. Part of this, Fleming (1992) suggests, is the need for a "joint process of critical reflection." Clearly in the situation as set out by Anderson and Elfert (1989) the Clinical Nurse Specialist is both a gatekeeper of autonomy and of control. Effective interventions require that Clinical Nurse Specialists examine their own feelings about dealing with these dilemmas, which may be beyond the remit of their role. If part of the educator role is to help the individual maintain a sense of control over their care, then they must be offered the opportunity, or be actively involved in decision making related to that care (Craig and Edwards, 1983).

DOES IT MAKE A DIFFERENCE?

The educator role presents an opportunity and a challenge for the Clinical Nurse Specialist. The opportunity is to demonstrate the impact of advanced nursing knowledge and skills within individualised packages of care. In many situations of chronic illness the Clinical Nurse Specialist is better placed than many medical practitioners to deal with the educational, social and psychological needs of individuals (Kerrison, 1990). The challenge is to illustrate, with evidence, the beneficial impact of the role, while remaining constantly mindful, that

> "So many patients do learn to master discomfort and treatment regimes without abdicating others' roles and sources of satisfaction."
> Wilson-Barnett and Batehup (1988)

The educator role can be both economic and efficient. However, one must ask the question: is it effective and does it make a difference? The call to demonstrate and document the benefits of patient education are growing (Smith, 1989). The need to develop evaluative methods which are themselves appropriate and effective should, as Youssef (1983) argues focus, on "patient outcomes to substantiate behavioural changes resulting from patient education." Effective health care is not just a case of giving people information about how care should be carried out, there must also be adequate resources (Anderson and Elfert, 1989).

Individuals demonstrating compliance could be seen as one measure of the effectiveness of the educator role, in that they are doing whatever it is they have been asked to do, but how effective is this in the long term? Another assumption is that the more people know, the more they will be able and willing to maintain an enhanced level of self-care. Clearly, it is rather optimistic to expect major lifestyle changes to occur as a consequence of short-term input, as the likelihood of effective change is greater overtime (Oberst, 1989). From Oberst's (1989) extensive review of the literature on patient education spanning the last 20 years, the conclusion was that while patient education worked, it appeared to be regardless of the strategies adopted. Indeed Mazzuca (1982) suggested that

"The standard presentation of medical facts and treatment rules are relatively ineffective in fostering the desired behaviour or helping people cope."

Consequently, there is a need to increase the sophistication of the measurement of effectiveness of patient education and movement towards the development of outcome measures that go beyond the assessment of knowledge, focusing on health gains for the individual and making clear the explicit contribution to the wider health of the nation. In many situations the skills of a Clinical Nurse Specialist are more appropriate than those of a medical practitioner. Indeed Bury (1991) in an examination of the sociology of chronic illness, suggested that there may be paradoxical expectations in the context of chronic illness, when medical intervention may be of limited effectiveness. Clinical Nurse Specialists are, therefore, uniquely positioned to utilise their close understanding of the individual's needs, thus enabling the construction of interventions specific and effective for that person.

The educator role may be practised in many settings, using a variety of strategies and approaches, from one-to-one, to systematic group teaching programmes. The skills of the Clinical Nurse Specialist are aimed at the assessment and planning of educational interventions which will assist the individuals to manage and meet their own health-care needs as far as possible. In many cases the Clinical Nurse Specialist is best equipped to facilitate this process, for as Kerrison (1990) suggests in relation to diabetic care: "education is now such an important part of diabetic work that investment of capital in special buildings dedicated to this is taking place." The educator role, therefore, consumes a considerable amount of the Clinical Nurse Specialist's resources, and given the wider demands for the evaluation of effectiveness there is a necessity to evaluate these educational interventions. Priest (1989), in discussing the evaluation of the educator role, suggests that adopting a structure, process and outcome approach may provide a useful framework for systematic evaluation.

The identification of the resources allocated to this role is an important first stage in demonstrating their impact. How much of the Clinical Nurse Specialist's time is spent on educational interventions? What approaches are used? How many teaching sessions are carried out and how many individuals are seen? Unless the amount of resources presently used to fulfil the role can be identified, it will be difficult to assess whether they are sufficient to bring about the desired effect.

However, this pre-supposes that there is a clear view of what is the desired effect. Clear identification of changes in health behaviours, and ultimately health-care outcomes, are possible through the systematic planning of an individual's care. Unless specific goals of care and interventions are identified jointly by the Clinical Nurse Specialist and the individual concerned, it will be impossible to evaluate effectiveness. Care-plans provide the evidence that on individual basis educational interventions have made a difference (Close, 1988). With such evidence it would be possible for the Clinical Nurse Specialist to evaluate on a wider scale the collective contribution made as an educator. Clearly, attempting to identify the specific contribution of the educational role is not an easy process, and it is a challenge that should not be ignored just because it is complex. Ingersoll (1988) suggested that attempts to identify specific outcomes related to the Clinical Nurse Specialist role, in its entirety, are difficult, but makes it clear that without valid and reliable documentation of interventions, the measurement of outcomes is difficult. The need to document the benefits of education for the individual is also emphasised by Smith (1989) who suggested that, not only should educational interventions enable the individual to "incorporate learned health behaviours into daily routines" but that "economic, physiologic, social and psychological benefits" of education should be captured. This desire to demonstrate the social consequences of the educator role of nurses generally was echoed by Oberst (1989), who went on to suggest that

"Selection of outcome measures needs to go beyond assessment of knowledge gains to include indicators of adherence to the self-care regimen and health outcomes."

Within health care generally the demands to demonstrate effectiveness are growing, and the Clinical Nurse Specialist as an educator operating within this context must be mindful of these wider pressures. The call to increase the sophistication of the measures of effectiveness within the Health Service clearly have consequences for the Clinical Nurse Specialist role (Morath, 1988; Bond and Thomas, 1991; Long, 1992). While the identification of outcomes specifically attributable to the educator role of the Clinical Nurse Specialist may be difficult, it presents a challenge which must be taken up. Bond and Thomas (1991), in their work on measuring the outcomes of nursing, argue that unless the specific contribution of nurses to health care is identified, it may remain invisible. This concern equally relates to the educator role of the Clinical Nurse Specialist, and Priest (1989) warns of the dangers ahead, by suggesting that attempting to evaluate the impact of the Clinical Nurse Specialist as an educator "is a more difficult indicator to measure, since changes in patient health status could be multifactorial in origin." An encouraging source of support for this process is the development and introduction of clinical audit in the National Health Service, assisting professionals to reflect upon the service they deliver in order to ensure effectiveness in terms of service delivery and professional accountability. The contribution of Clinical Nurse Specialists to this process is not insignificant, and using the bio-psycho-social model, they are able to facilitate a holistic approach to the analysis of both individual and service outcomes. Their contribution must include an understanding of the significance of educator role.

So far, the discussion has focused on evaluating the effectiveness of the educator role in relation to recipients of care, but it is evident that the Clinical Nurse Specialist is a corporate resource, and as such has an educational role with the staff of the organisation. Through the continuing development and education of staff within the organisation, the Clinical Nurse Specialist is able not only to influence the quality of direct nursing care, but also the indirect care of individuals by the organisation. To facilitate this process Priest (1989) advocates that the Clinical Nurse Specialists collaborate with staff development departments. While the concept of Clinical Nurse Specialists as a corporate resource was explored by McDougall (1987) who identified the contribution they can make to organisational development as a form of internal consultant, the value of this contribution was that

"The Clinical Nurse Specialists are an asset since they understand organisational structures as well as interpersonal dynamics. Thus, these consultants can assist management in assessing, diagnosing, and identifying strengths and weaknesses of the organisation's structural and/or behavioural processes such as work flow, interpersonal relations, communications and intergroup relations needing improvement."

McDougall (1987)

In many instances the Clinical Nurse Specialist is able to act as a catalyst, encouraging collaborative working across professional groups, thus providing a cohesive service, not only for the benefit of the individuals who need it, but also for the organisation as a whole.

Previous discussion has focused on whether the educator role makes a difference for individuals and organisations. The question that remains to be addressed is: how does the individual Clinical Nurse Specialist review their own contribution as an educator in relation to other Clinical Nurse Specialists?

PEER REVIEW

For Clinical Nurse Specialists it is imperative that they maintain credibility, and in order to do so they must attend to their own educational development, and one mechanism which is increasingly being used for this is peer review. In Chapter 1 the concern about the uneven development of Clinical Nurse Specialist posts was explored, and while this situation may present difficulties, it also presents opportunities. One such opportunity is that of peer support and review, to enable the growth of the role. Such an approach would enable Clinical Nurse Specialists working in a diversity of areas to identify generic issues, such as the educator role, and to share examples of good practice. At the same time such a strategy would provide Clinical Nurse Specialists, who could find themselves in an isolated position, with a valuable source of professional support. At present there are a number of national professional groups catering for the needs of Clinical Nurse Specialists working in particular fields. However these are external to the employees' organisation and it may well be that the establishment of a peer review network, within an organisation, would assist the process of contributing not only to the corporate goals, but ultimately to the quality of care.

The educator role of the Clinical Nurse Specialist is probably the most influential role in making a difference to individuals' health-related behaviour. On the wider scale the Clinical Nurse Specialist needs constantly to develop skills in empowering individuals to take on such responsibilities, while at the same time developing methodologies to evaluate the effectiveness of educational interventions. The publication of *The Health of the Nation* (Department of Health, 1991) provides an excellent opportunity for Clinical Nurse Specialists to demonstrate the contribution they make as educators for health.

REFERENCES

Altschul A. (1983) The consumer's voice: nursing implications. *Journal of Advanced Nursing*, 8(3): 175–183.

Anderson J.M. and Elfert H. (1989) Managing chronic illness in the family: women as caretakers. *Journal of Advanced Nursing*, 14(2): 735–743.

Antonovsky A. (1992) Janforum: locus of control theory. *Journal of Advanced Nursing*, 17(8): 1014–1015.

Ashworth P.D., Longmate M.A. and Morrison P. (1992) Patient participation: its meaning and significance in the context of caring. *Journal of Advanced Nursing*, 17: 1430–1439.

Bond S. and Thomas L. (1991) Issues in measuring outcomes of nursing. *Journal of Advanced Nursing*, 16(12): 1492–1502.

Bury M. (1991) The sociology of chronic illness: a review of research and prospects. *Sociology of Health and Illness*, 13(4): 451–456.

Close A. (1988) Patient education: a literature review. *Journal of Advanced Nursing*, 13(2): 203–213.

Craig H.M. and Edwards J.E. (1983) Adaptation in chronic illness: an eclectic model for nurses. *Journal of Advanced Nursing*, 8(5): 379–404.

Davidhizar R. (1983) Critique of the health-belief model. *Journal of Advanced Nursing*, 8(6): 467–472.

Department of Health (1991) *The Health of the Nation: A Strategy for Health in England, Cm1523*. HMSO, London.

Dracup K. and Meleis A. (1982) Compliance: an interactionalist approach. *Nursing Research*, 31(1): 31–36.

Fleming V.E.M. (1992) Client education: a futuristic outlook. *Journal of Advanced Nursing*, 17: 158–163.

Ingersoll G.L. (1988) Evaluating the input of a Clinical Nurse Specialist. *Clinical Nurse Specialist*, 2(3): 150–155.

Jarvis P. (1983) *Professional Education*. Croom Helm, London.

Kerrison S. (1990) A diplomat in the job: diabetes nursing and the changing division of labour in diabetic care. *Health and Social Services Research Unit Research Paper*, 4 January, South Bank Polytechnic, London.

Long A.F. (1992) Evaluating health services: from value for money to valuing of health services. In Pollitt C. and Harrison S. (Eds), *Handbook of Public Services Management*. Blackwell, Oxford.

Mazzuca S.A. (1982) Does patient education in chronic disease have therapeutic value? *Journal of Chronic Disease*, 35(7): 521–529.

McDougall G.J. (1987) The role of the Clinical Nurse Specialist consultant in organizational development. *Clinical Nurse Specialist*, 1(3): 133–139.

Morath J.M. (1988) The Clinical Nurse Specialist: evaluation issues. *Nursing Management*, 19(3): 72–80.

Oberst M.J. (1989) Perspectives on research in patient teaching. *Nursing Clinics of North America*, 24(3): 621–628.

Orem D. (1991) *Nursing: Concepts of Practice*, 4th edn. Mosby, St. Louis, Missouri.

Pollitt C. (1984) The state and health care. In McLennan G., Held D. and Hall S. (Eds), *State and Society in Contemporary Britain: A Critical Introduction*. Polity Press, Cambridge.

Priest A-R. (1989) The Clinical Nurse Specialist as educator. In Hamic A.B. and Spross J.A. (Eds), *The Clinical Nurse Specialist in Theory and Practice*, 2nd edn. Saunders, Philadelphia, Pennsylvania.

Smith C.E. (1989) Overview of patient education: opportunities and challenges for the 21st century. *Nursing Clinics of North America*, 24(3): 583–587.

Waterworth S. and Luker K. (1990) Reluctant collaborators: do patients want to be involved in decisions concerning care? *Journal of Advanced Nursing*, 15(8): 971–976.

Wilson-Barnett J. and Batehup L. (1988) *Patient Problems: A Research Base for Nursing Care*. Scutari, London.

Wilson-Barnett J. and Fordham M. (1982) *Recovery from Illness*. Wiley, Chichester.

Youssef F.A. (1983) Compliance with therapeutic regimens: a follow up study for patients with affective disorders. *Journal of Advanced Nursing*, 8(6): 513–517.

CHAPTER FIVE

The law and ethics: the graveyard of nurse specialism?

Caroline Soar

The nature of nurse specialism is diverse, and role functions within the same specialisms differ from employer to employer. As clinical knowledge increases so the Clinical Nurse Specialist's role increases so that practitioners are taking on more and more, and issues of accountability and professionalism are no longer clearly demarked. A potential minefield of legal and ethical problems awaits the nurse specialist. Graveyards, as the title shows, are full of not just those who have died, but also full of grief. Graveyards are also full of epitaphs cast in tablets of stone, final messages to people and while the epitaph is final it can be open to question. The law is akin to an epitaph, while ethics lay the law open to question.

Nurses have a strong sense of justice, and aptly distinguish between right and wrong, fairness and unfairness. This is the subjective self, the moral conscience, from which nurses determine the ethical stance they take. Having a sense of justice and knowing about the law is not the same thing. However, there are some nurses who still remain somewhat ignorant of the law as it governs their practice. This ignorance exists for a variety of reasons, and experience shows that the most common is lack of education in this area. The second reason is that as professionals, nurses do not like unfairness and may in some circumstances seek to avoid it. Sometimes the law seems very unfair and very uncaring in meting out justice. We need not look far; take the court case involving a Consultant who administered a lethal dose of potassium chloride to a patient in intractable pain. The legal system found the Consultant guilty of manslaughter and punished him in a manner appropriately determined for the 'crime' committed. To some health care professionals, that may seem totally unfair, and we may believe that because the intention was to relieve suffering, the action was right, and find the Consultant not guilty. No matter how emotive nurses' arguments may be in defence of his conduct, the fact is that he broke the law and as a consequence he was punished. This is not meant to encourage defensive practice by discussing the legal and ethical issues, for if nurses were that ignorant of the law they would probably not be practising today. However, law cannot be left to the lawyers, medicine to doctors and nursing to nurses. The law affects us all, and health care professionals have a duty to understand how it affects them. For example, when driving a car it would be no defence in a court of law to say that you drove at 60 mph through a 30 mph zone because your nursing training did not include a session on the Road Traffic Act. If all professionals were to blinker themselves in their own profession without understanding how other professions impinge upon them, then they would certainly end up in the graveyard. Indeed, Tingle (1990) in his articles on Nurses and The Law, states "Ignorance of the law does not excuse" and Dimond (1990) states that "Accountability is steeped in legal issues. Law cannot be left to the lawyers." If emotive arguments are used to defend actions, nurses must accept that emotiveness and the law do not make compatible bedfellows, and as a result accept the consequences.

An example of this which is a common occurrence in nursing, is deciding, no matter how ill a nurse might feel, not to go off sick. The work area is busy and no matter how unwell, the nurse feels that by going off sick patients would be disappointed. There is a very busy day ahead and support staff are already off sick, so the nurse decides to go to work and struggle on. During the course of the day the nurse makes a mistake, and as a result, a patient suffers damage. Later on the nurse learns that the patient is going to sue. During the ensuing enquiry, all the mitigating circumstances are included in the plea of defence, however the employing Authority or Trust refuses to cover the nurse because the sickness policy was not adhered to.

No matter what the emotive argument, the bitter pill to swallow is that on the day in question, the nurse soldiered on to the best of ability, only to feel totally rejected and hard-done-by when sympathy and understanding were needed. Yet the employing authority is quite within its rights: it is not concerned with the emotive arguments, but with the adherence to its policies. Policies are an employing authority's safeguard, and ensure that its employees do not stray from the legal requirements laid down in statute which policies seek to put into operation.

In law, two types of liability apply to Health Authorities: direct liability which means that if something goes wrong the Authority itself is at fault, and vicarious or indirect liability whereby the Authority is responsible for the faults or civil wrongs of others. Therefore, an employer is liable for all an employee's civil wrongs provided the employee is on duty at the time of the wrong, is working within the parameters of the job description and contract, and adheres to the policies, procedures, guidelines and protocols laid down by the employer. An employer may waive the right to cover the employee if the above conditions are not adhered to.

At the beginning of the chapter, it was suggested that as knowledge and skills increase, the role of the Clinical Nurse Specialist increases and practitioners are taking on more in terms of workload. In order for Clinical Nurse Specialists to ensure that they have the employer covering liability, contracts and job descriptions must be made explicit so that both the employer and the Clinical Nurse Specialist have a clear understanding of what the specialist is permitted to do.

To give an example of this, if Clinical Nurse Specialists have been given permission by a medical colleague to alter drug doses if they feel the situation warrants it, and nowhere is this written down in a job description, policy or procedure, then they need to check with their employer that they are covered to undertake this role, even if they know they are competent to do so. This is one part of the Clinical Nurse Specialist's accountability.

To be accountable is to be answerable for the care a nurse gives and the service a nurse offers. To do this, Clinical Nurse Specialists need to understand what their duty of care is. Inherent in accountability is the need to maintain high standards of practice, and Dimond (1990) cites four areas in which health professionals are accountable. The Clinical Nurse Specialist is answerable to the patient and society via the civil or criminal courts, to the employer through contract, and to the profession via the Conduct Committee at the United Kingdom Central Council for Nurses, Midwives and Health Visitors. To be professionally accountable means that nurses are answerable for their actions while their name is on the professional register. The point of conduct here is that they need not be on duty to be answerable for their actions. There have been cases where nurses have found themselves in court for offences which have nothing to do with nursing. Society via the Criminal Court and the profession via the Conduct Committee are entitled to judge the case. The profession has the right to expect reasonable behaviour at all times from its professionals in order that public trust and confidence are upheld. Therefore, nurses are under obligation not only to provide a duty of care, but to behave in a manner appropriate to their profession even when they are off duty, and society has the right to expect nurses to answer for their actions. Rae (1987) states that:

"The legal duty of care encompasses the professional, moral, ethical and sociological duties of care within which nursing operates."

Realistically, nurses must not blinker themselves to what is just legal and professional, they need to accept that they have a duty to understand their moral duty of care, their ethical duty of care and their sociological duty of care.

What then is the moral and ethical duty of care for the Clinical Nurse Specialist? The distinction between morals and ethics is made by Tschudin (1986) who claims that morals concerns itself with threats to be forestalled and ethics concerns itself with ideals to be pursued.

To illustrate this, the role of the health educator and promoter is part of every Clinical Nurse Specialist's job, and one of the objectives of *The Health of The Nation* (Department of Health, 1991) is to reduce cigarette smoking. The moral approach using Tschudin's (1986) distinction is concerned with the health risks smoking causes and the ethical approach concentrates on promoting taking responsibility for one's own health care. This distinction can be taken further and Tschudin (1986) distinguishes between normative and descriptive ethics. Normative ethics in health care pursues the concepts of health, rights of patients, dimensions of caring and concepts such as compassion and commitment. They are traditionally the concern of nurses, and raise holistic/broad questions, while descriptive ethics in health care pursues the psychology of illness, physiology of stress and social pressures in chronic disease. They are traditionally the concern of doctors and raise more focused questions.

Clinical Nurse Specialists will therefore ask the question: Should the patient receive a specific form of treatment while doctors are concerned with how the patient will receive this treatment? Normative ethics are usually accompanied by codes which state how people should behave, for example, *The Scope of Professional Practice for Nurses, Midwives and Health Visitors* (UKCC, 1992b) or the *Declaration of Helsinki* (World Medical Association, 1964) which deals with recommendations to guide doctors in biomedical research involving human subjects.

Using this distinction in practice, potential ethical problems may arise. The Clinical Nurse Specialist will be concerned with concepts and questions about health, patients' rights, and make suggestions to the multi-disciplinary team as to how we should behave ethically in these situations. The doctor might on the other hand be concerned with the analysis of illness and the curing of disease, and rather than recommend how we should behave, will emphasise what we should obscure. A doctor in a rush to find a cure may compromise the value system of the Clinical Nurse Specialist who may not agree with the treatment and the way we behave toward the patient while finding the cure. The problem is an ethical one, a possible solution is a skill-based one.

ASSERTIVENESS AND NEGOTIATION

Again experience suggests, when addressing the legal and ethical issues of consent, some patients are being given information about their operation, and the consent form is being written so ambiguously, that it gives surgeons open licence to do what they regard as necessary. If nurses were more assertive, this practice could cease. If Clinical Nurse Specialism is about enhancing our practice and our advanced education, the fundamental question to pose is: Do nurses know what our normative ethical viewpoint is and what duty of care arises out of this? If nurses do know, are they harming their patients because they are wary about arguing, or have no channels open to them to argue from their normative stance with medical colleagues? If this is so, from what basis are Clinical Nurse Specialists stating that they are Clinical Nurse Specialists?

One avenue open to them is the *Code of Professional Conduct* (UKCC, 1992a) which should provide the means to enhance professional accountability, and empowers them to fulfil the role of patient advocate. However, advocacy by definition is relatively easy to understand. The *Oxford English Dictionary* states that "an advocate is one who supports or speaks in favour of, one who pleads for another."

Nurses constantly take on new concepts in nursing in attempting to improve patient care; some examples are holistic care, the named nurse and patient advocacy. Nurses ascribe to these beliefs but what personal and professional price might they have to pay to implement them? Nurses need to take account of the implications of what they state they ascribe to. Returning then to a legal duty to care, nurses find they are bound by *The Nurses, Midwives and Health Visitors Acts, 1979* and *1992*, and *The Nurses, Midwives and Health Visitors Rules Approval Order 1983 Statutory Instrument No. 873*, which requires, among other things, that the nurse assess, plan, implement and evaluate care. Nowhere is it stated that nurses are mandated to use a model of nursing, yet if the legal duty of care encompasses the ethical duty, then values must be made explicit in the model of care used. The model of nursing used is a reflection of values. The choice of model used, be it Roper *et al.* (1985), Orem (1991), Peplau (1991) or an eclectic model, must enable the nurse and the patient to enter into a relationship which acknowledges and respects the patient as having rights and needs. The model should clearly show who, within the relationship, is responsible for what, and when the Clinical Nurse Specialist should act as patient advocate.

If Clinical Nurse Specialists do not use a model of nursing, and work closely with medical colleagues, then perhaps they ascribe to a continuation of a medical model used by medical colleagues when assessing patients. There are potential legal and ethical problems with this. Firstly, Clinical Nurse Specialists are not qualified to use a medical model, and secondly, unless extended role training has been undertaken for specific tasks, they are not competent to use it. Therefore, to adhere to these value statements made, Clinical Nurse Specialists must value patients from a nursing perspective. This is difficult unless they value nursing as a specialism, and it seems impossible to be answerable if they have not considered the nature and implications of professional accountability, patient advocacy and nursing values.

Part of the Clinical Nurse Specialists' accountability function is to provide the patient with a high standard of nursing care for which they must be answerable. Forms of liability arise in cases of negligence, which is one of the most frequent type of case to come before the courts in health care practice. Negligence has to be proved on three counts: firstly, a nurse owed a duty of care to a patient; secondly, there had been a breach of that duty; and thirdly, as a result of the breach, the patient had suffered damage. Negligent behaviour can be by act, omission and inappropriate delegation. Standards are not only addressed in nursing, but also addressed in law and centre on the notion of falling short of the required professional standard. In cases of negligence, the required professional standard is weighed up and deemed actionable if it causes the patient harm. Some areas to consider in practice will now be explored.

COMMUNICATING WITH PATIENTS

What would constitute negligence in this area? If Clinical Nurse Specialists imparted wrong information that resulted in damage, or gave nursing advice to someone who is not one of their patients, say, for example, a person who happens to know their neighbour is a nurse, then this constitutes negligence.

Physical damage is more easily recognisable than psychological damage, but the areas become blurred for Clinical Nurse Specialists working with therapies such as psychotherapy or counselling, and the client should be fully informed of the nature and possible effect of the therapy. Information should not be withheld from a patient, for example about possible side-effects of a treatment that may result in damage.

OBEYING INSTRUCTIONS

If Clinical Nurse Specialists are asked to carry out procedures they do not feel competent to do, then they must make this known to the appropriate authority. This ties in with extending the role. Even if a Clinical Nurse Specialist knows they are competent to extend their role but considers it unsafe to do so on this occasion for whatever reason, they should not extend their role if it has the potential to harm patients.

LACK OF EXPERIENCE

Unfortunately there are some areas of nurse specialism where education to prepare nurses for their specialist role is still lacking. One moment they are nurses with some knowledge, the next moment they have the title of Clinical Nurse Specialist and are expected to give specialist advice. If this is the situation, then nurses must adhere to clause 4 of the *Code of Professional Conduct* (UKCC, 1992a) which states that

"You must acknowledge any limitations in your knowledge and competence and decline any duties or responsibilities unless able to perform them in a safe and skilled manner."

Perhaps a task to undertake is to ask ourself: Are our standards of care clearly defined, safe and measurable? Are they commensurate with our philosophy of care and what is our minimal acceptable standard? These issues should be encompassed in quality assurance programmes which are a prerequisite of the *NHS and Community Care Act 1990* (Department of Health, 1990). When stating that quality is everybody's business, it is not just National Health Service business, but the business of the courts too. Thus we ensure that patients are protected against unsafe practices.

CONSENT

The next consideration is the law of consent. Dimond (1990) in outlining the basic principles, states that any adult, mentally competent person has the right in law to consent to any touching of their person. Consent takes two forms, tacit or implied consent, and actual or real consent. Tacit or implied means that the patient by virtue of being present in the consulting room or clinic is consenting, whereas actual or real consent is consent made in writing, the most common type of this form of consent being the patient's signature on an appropriate consent form. Problems, both legal and ethical arise with each.

Consider implied consent, where, for example, a person who is newly diagnosed as diabetic agrees to an appointment with a Clinical Nurse Specialist in a clinic. What is this person consenting to? Many Clinical Nurse Specialists may think the person is consenting to treatment but this is not the case. What they are consenting to is assessment. Furthermore they are consenting to a particular type of assessment because of the nature of the Clinical Nurse Specialist role. The person therefore is consenting to a nursing assessment. This again, is another reason for Clinical Nurse Specialists to have a clear view of what the role entails. It would be impossible to undertake a high standard of nursing assessment if Clinical Nurse Specialists were unsure what their nursing role entailed.

This assessment having been carried out, before any treatment can be agreed, the person will need to know the outcome of the assessment and proposed plan of care in order to make an informed choice when consenting to the treatment suggested. Dimond (1990) states that as far as the law is concerned there is no specific requirement that consent for treatment should be given in any particular way. All are equally valid, but the emphasis of the value lies in the proof that consent was given.

True consent should be fully informed consent. However, what does informed consent mean? How 'informed' should informed consent be? The principle of beneficence, that is doing good, should be uppermost in the Clinical Nurse Specialist's value system, and an ethical question arises out of this in relation to consent. Will telling the patient all the effects and side-effects of the treatment harm them rather than do them good? The principle of beneficence needs to be weighed against the principle of non-maleficence, that is the principle of not doing harm. The aim at best should be to strive to do good, and at least to strive to do no harm.

In law, whether consent is tacit or real, there is what is known as the prudent patient test. This means that if patients have the intelligence or competence to understand the nature, purpose and effects of the treatment, and this should include the side-effects of the treatment, then they should be fully informed. This has ethical implications and may place the Clinical Nurse Specialist in a compromising position. How much should the Clinical Nurse Specialist tell the patient? What is needed is to weigh up what is reasonable and of benefit to the patient from a nursing point of view. To do this Clinical Nurse Specialists need to know what competence might mean.

A patient is competent if able fully to understand the nature, purpose and effects of the treatment and the consequences of receiving the treatment or of refusing it. Competent patients therefore are able to make fully informed decisions about the health care they receive; this is one way of respecting the patient as an autonomous individual. Good communication between both nurse specialist and patient is vital here. With implied consent patients might non-verbally indicate they are willing to accept treatment, for example, rolling up a sleeve for an injection. However the Clinical Nurse Specialist needs to ensure verbally that it is still permissible to administer the injection because the patient could think it was the blood pressure that was going to be measured.

How free and autonomous should Clinical Nurse Specialists allow patients to be, and at what stage for the benefit of the individual should the Clinical Nurse Specialist intervene in order to prevent harm? Autonomy is also about empowering and if we empower the patient, we should also have empowerment. In society today, no individual is totally free to practise autonomously. This is because as professionals we have a duty to adhere to the law, the social moral codes and our professional codes. Yet if we give a patient true autonomy we could legally compromise ourselves. As professionals we profess to know best, that is how society views us and the law judges us.

Most patients would like to make decisions about their care and treatment, but also they look to the professional for guidance and advice. To leave the decisions totally to the patient might mean they lose all confidence in the professional, or think that the professional lacks the knowledge to practise. Consent and autonomy are about good verbal interaction between patient and nurse specialist, ensuring that adequate professional advice and guidance are available to the patient.

CONFIDENTIALITY

Confidentiality is another issue where law and ethics may be at odds with each other. Can our patients trust us to keep a confidence? To what extent are we duty bound to keep that confidence? Like a priest, the power of the confessional is an essential part of our role. Yet it is like a colander full of holes and because of the legal implications the ethical principle cannot be absolute.

The patient has a right to privacy, to feel safe in trusting the nurse specialist. However, the reality is that the patient, professional and State can all lay claim to a patient's confidences. A broad example here is the notification of infectious diseases, and notification of drug addiction. Ultimately the records kept by the Health Authority are the property of the Secretary of State for Health, and as a matter of law patients may be entitled to look at them should the need arise. Clinical Nurse Specialists working in the community who use patient-held records need to ensure that they have a copy of the records. Should the records be required in a court of law and the notes have been mislaid, then all Clinical Nurse Specialists can rely upon is their memory. This is especially important because a person has three years to take legal action for damages if something goes wrong, or three years within the knowledge of something going wrong to take legal action.

ETHICS AND RESEARCH

Another area of ethical concern is that of research and research trials. Nursing, in order to advance knowledge to enhance practice must rely upon the research process, and research by the very nature of what it aims to do is full of unknowns. If Clinical Nurse Specialists agree to help out with clinical trials they may find they face ethical problems with the use of placebos or the new treatment being tested. The *Declaration of Helsinki* (World Medical Association, 1964) emphasises that all subjects to experimentation must give informed consent, as was discussed earlier in this chapter. The declaration goes on to state that if the doctor considers it essential not to obtain informed consent, the specific reason for this proposal should be stated in the experimentation protocol for transmission to the independent committees. Our medical colleagues, like all other health-care professionals, are concerned with doing the best they can for their patients. A potential problem here is the question of what is best. This is where the Clinical Nurse Specialist may have a difference of opinion with medical colleagues. If Clinical Nurse Specialists identify harm being done as a result of research trials, they must make known their concerns. They may not be in a position to comment on the medical aspects of the research trials because they may feel unqualified to do so. However, they must voice their concerns on the protocols of the experimentation if they consider the research is doing more harm than considered necessary, or that had the patient been fully informed, they would not have agreed to the trials.

At the beginning of this chapter, it was suggested that the law is like an epitaph cast in tablets of stone and ethics lay the law open to question. All Health Authorities have an Ethics Committee whose key function is to determine protocols for research. Research is only one aspect of the ethical issues, problems and dilemmas which face us in our day-to-day practice. It is important that nurses should have a forum to express their ethical concerns, and in some Health Authority nurses have set up ethics interest groups to air these issues.

This chapter has touched on the broad legal issues that affect Clinical Nurse Specialists today. The ethical issues which arise from legislation or lack of it must ensure that professionals question practice. Before claiming clinical competence at a specialist level, Clinical Nurse Specialists must be clinically confident that the morality of their practice makes them clinically credible. A concluding suggestion is that if Clinical Nurse Specialists are unsure about any aspect of their practice, they identify the appropriate local channels and ask for the correct advice and guidance.

REFERENCES

Department of Health (1990) *The National Health Service and Community Care Act 1990*. HMSO, London.

Department of Health (1991) *The Health of the Nation: A Strategy for Health in England, Cm 1523*. HMSO, London.

DHSS (1979) *The Nurses, Midwives and Health Visitors Act 1979*. HMSO, London.

Dimond B. (1990) *Legal Aspects of Nursing*. Prentice-Hall, Hemel Hempstead.

Orem D. (1991) *Nursing: Concepts of Practice*, 4th edn. Mosby, St Louis, Missouri.

Peplau H. (1991) *Interpersonal Theory in Nursing Practice*. Macmillan, London.

Rae K. (1987) Negligence. Nursing, Vol. 3, No. 14. (February) In Holland S. (1991) *Accountability in Health Visiting: A Pack for Returners, Practitioners and Managers*. Health Visitors Association, London.

Roper N., Logan W. and Tierney A. (1985) *The Elements of Nursing*, 2nd edn. Churchill Livingstone, Edinburgh.

Tingle J. (1990) Nurses and the laws: a hard lesson ... medical and nursing negligence. *Nursing Times*, 87(9): 44–45.

Tschudin V. (1986) *Ethics in Nursing*. Heinemann Nursing, London.

United Kingdom Central Council (1992a) *Code of Professional Conduct*. UKCC, London.

United Kingdom Central Council (1992b) *The Scope of Professional Practice for Nurses, Midwives and Health Visitors*. UKCC, London.

World Medical Association (1964) *Declaration of Helsinki*. World Medical Association, Geneva.

CHAPTER SIX

Evaluating the impact: using a business planning approach

Sarah Smart

PUTTING EVALUATION IN CONTEXT: WHY BOTHER?

There may be a number of reasons why Clinical Nurse Specialists are concerned with the evaluation of their role. On the one hand, it may be about justifying the role and its expenditure against a perceived threat of reduction in services. On the other hand, it may be about taking the opportunity to develop the role and its place within the provider unit, and thus attract extra resources. No doubt the perspective will depend on the forces within individual units, however, using this chapter purely as a response to a threat may tend to limit its horizons. It is proposed that evaluation should be seen as an opportunity to stand back and examine the services currently offered, and identify what is still required.

There can be no doubt that the changing dynamics of health care have demanded a radical re-think of service provision, and that now is the time to achieve a new direction for Clinical Nurse Specialists' services. So often, a new role is started with a clear perception of what is required and two years down the road the specialist has become so absorbed with the mechanics of the job that sight of the overall plan has been lost. Time after time it is all too easy to respond to the demands of the clinical workload, following well known tramlines rather than carving a new path. Sometimes the energy invested in the job means that the best that can be done is to hurtle from one end of the week to the next extracting what satisfaction there is from direct patient contact.

Although this may feel comfortable, it is not the way to proceed. Now is the time to put the role on a concrete business footing as well as a clinical footing to ensure that it remains a key feature of all provider units' service mix.

CARVING THE PATH

Carving a new path could be very easy if the individual Clinical Nurse Specialists had only to consider themselves, the client group and immediate colleagues. No doubt Clinical Nurse Specialists would wish that their objectives could be achieved in spite of others. The reality is of course quite different, and it is not just a question of defining objectives according to the perceptions of the nurse and trying to link them to medical colleagues – a task difficult enough in itself. Now there are wider considerations related to meeting the expectations of all consumers, internal and external, as well as purchasers. All of a sudden it has become essential to understand the requirements of others, and to define the service in relation to these requirements explicitly. Finally, there is the real challenge, that of helping purchasers understand what could be provided and where they have not recognised a potential service, to sell it to them, getting the Clinical Nurse Specialists' objectives on to the purchaser's agenda.

To many health care professionals, this radical change may be perceived as strange and contrary to previous work ethics and practice. This chapter cannot, in itself, reduce the anxiety associated with such a fundamental change. Instead it attempts to define the new rules of the game and guide the movement of the key players. There is a deliberate concentration on defining objectives, as a service cannot be evaluated against a blank sheet selecting standards and measurements from thin air. If this is all that is required, the specialist could trawl the literature for measurements and avoid reading the rest of this chapter. Equally, it is suggested that an over-emphasis on the writing of detailed standards rather misses the point and expends energy in, initially at least, the wrong direction. It may be that defining the structure, process and outcome components of standards is a useful internal mechanism for checking performance, although sometimes the content of such standards precludes meaningful and frequent evaluation, and such an approach may not provide consumers and purchasers with what they require. It is proposed instead that one line indicators of performance are defined which explicitly demonstrate that purchaser requirements are being met. Such indicators should be capable of more routine monitoring with further detail added later in the form of policies or standards, should more guidance be required as to how such indicators will be achieved and maintained.

DEFINING THE BENCHMARK: EVALUATING THE IMPACT AGAINST WHAT?

The benchmark is the standard desired for a section of the client population. In this situation, the client can be a range of people from patients to internal and external customers such as General Practitioners (GPs), but it is perhaps more straightforward and indeed correct to start from the patient's perspective. Be warned however against resting here; the melting pot of benchmarks encompasses all purchasers and a comprehensive range of requirements will need to be defined.

The building blocks of benchmarks can be considered (Figure 6.1) as follows:

Roof	Professional Requirements (keeping the rain out)
First floor	External customer expectations (cannot be built before the foundations and first floor)
Ground floor	Internal customer expectations (don't be tempted to build a bungalow)
Foundations	Patients' expectations (the more effort spent here, the stronger the house)

In order to lay the foundations, the site must first be surveyed. There are two start points: examining what is currently provided or starting right at the beginning by examining what the client group needs/wants. The author would advocate the latter approach, as it builds in the justifi-

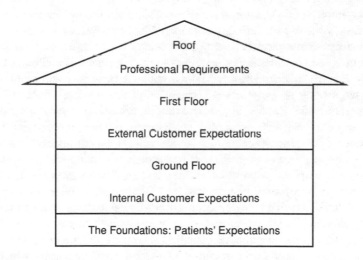

Figure 6.1   *The building blocks of benchmarks*

cation for the service right the way through, rather than just saying that a part of the service is on offer because it has always been there.

Foundations: patients' expectations

Defining the scope of the patient group is essential as the specialist's objectives will be quite different depending on whether the requirements centre on the whole of the client population, or just a select group. This first step should be done in conjunction with the question: what is the service trying to achieve for this group? For instance: is the Clinical Nurse Specialist trying to achieve the end product of:

1. All diabetic patients who come into contact with acute services will have access to nursing staff trained in diabetic management or
2. Patients having difficulty in coming to terms with their diabetic management will have access to an individual support programme to facilitate adaption?

It is unlikely that the service can achieve both to the same degree unless the specialist has an unusually large department. The objectives are substantially different as the first offers something for everyone, the second a lot for a few, and some degree of prioritisation is required. It is vital not to limit this stage by looking at the services currently provided. Instead, have a view of the grand plan – the complete scope of what is required for the client group.

The importance and indeed the difficulty of this first step cannot be over-emphasised. A vast number of possibilities exist and there will be a need to go to the literature to assess what objectives are reasonable and achievable. Past records held by the Clinical Nurse Specialist may be useful to assess which approaches seemed to offer the best outcomes but new investigative studies directly involving the consumer will probably be required. It is likely that the patient will have a complex mixture of expectations which are subject to different influences. Although simple comparison with US research is not recommended, some findings are clearly applicable. Wilson (1988) identifies that consumer decision making is subject to both internal and external influences such as perception of the situation, motives and personality in the case of the former and life style, demographic variables and social class in the latter. It follows that as well as consumer requirements being influenced in such ways, the ability of the patient to verbalise expectations will be similarly affected. Defining expectations demands of the patient an ability to describe thoughts and meanings and any given person may be no more able to explain and describe these than anyone else; vocabulary may be poverty stricken and the perspective may be too difficult to comprehend (Shatzman and Strauss, 1973).

Despite the difficulty in helping patients to voice their expectations, this research is essential as it cannot be assumed that nurses will inherently provide what the patient requires. Although frequently, consumer satisfaction is assumed to increase as the quality of care increases (Carter and Mowad, 1988), the opposite has been found. Eriksen (1987) found an inverse relationship between the two and that patient satisfaction increased with the amount of social courtesy and service extended, and that this was not always reflective of the quality of care given. Carter and Mowad (1988) suggest an interesting comparison with the airline industry:

"A passenger disembarking from a plane rarely lauds the airline for a safe arrival. Rather, he or she focuses on the quality of the food or the speed with which the luggage arrives. Patients leaving hospital expect to recover from their operation. Their recollection of their hospital stay centres around the courtesy of personnel, the cleanliness of the room, and the temperature of the food."

Difficult though this first step is, a number of possibilities should emerge:

1. The service provided matches the requirements of the patient.
2. The service fundamentally fails to address the requirements of the patient.
3. Patients have certain expectations that cannot be realised within current capabilities and resources.
4. All the services required are out there, but are fragmented.

The process of identification is time consuming, but pooling resources with Clinical Nurse Specialist colleagues with help from structured consumer voices like Community Health Councils will help make the task easier. There may indeed be a spin-off from such work in terms of role definition. Smith (1990) suggests that

"A further possibility for determining the use of the Clinical Nurse Specialist is to base the post on the demands made on the service and the key elements of the role. The essence of this idea is to consider placing the emphasis on the role components that best meet the demands placed on the service."

To take a stronger view, the role must be developed according to the demands placed upon it by the client group.

Following this first stage, the specialists should have at their disposal a range of patient-centred objectives that fulfil most expectations. The stairs can now be climbed to the first floor.

Ground floor: internal customer expectations

Although a clear understanding of the expectations of patients ensures a solid foundation, it does not in itself provide a complete picture of what is required from the Clinical Nurse Specialist service. Understanding the requirements of the local provider unit is vital to ensure that the needs of the internal customer are met and that the nurse specialist is on the units agenda with a solid place in the overall plan of services. The service expected may already be defined in broad terms by the senior management team and will be influenced by the unit's goals for the future, its quality/marketing objectives and plans for resource allocation.

The Clinical Nurse Specialists need to determine whether their services are seen as a key component and integral part of the unit's plan, or as a marginal, somewhat vulnerable offering. Gaining the internal customer's perspective is a difficult process particularly if the specialist encompasses the wider view, that is, across the acute/community boundary. With so many potential internal customers, an analysis of the key stake-holders is essential to ensure objectives are prioritised. Stakeholder analysis helps to identify the key customers with influence in the organisation: those that ultimately will affect the direction and achievement of objectives (Johnson and Scholes, 1988; Kakabadse *et al.*, 1988).

So what then are the requirements of the internal customer? Do they want a Macmillan nurse on call 24 hours a day, or every member of the medical staff kept up-to-date with the latest techniques in pain control? Do they just want to know the specialist's contact point, or know the criteria for referral? How do they see the service placed and how do they wish the service to be developed? Giving the internal customer the opportunity to define the specialist's objectives is preferable to lobbying colleagues to support something they are not sure they want; inappropriate especially if they pay towards the costs of the service. Offering customers a say in what is provided ensures that the relationship with the specialist is cemented and that the service commands support.

First floor: external purchases

The requirements of district purchasers/commissioning teams and GP fund-holders will have a major influence on the specialist's objectives.

The power of these customers should not be underestimated as at the end of the day the provider does not have a service unless someone is willing to pay for it, and never assume that the purchaser has to continue to buy the same type and volume of service as that previously offered. If external customers have a choice of where to buy, it can be presumed that they will make decisions based on the ability of that provider to meet their objectives. Working with the purchasers now to meet their requirements will put the specialist in a strong position both to maintain and in future to develop the service.

The external customer's agenda is gaining in strength and focus with national direction from the *Patients' Charter* (Department of Health, 1991b) and *The Health of the Nation* (Department of Health, 1991a) initiatives, as well as analysis of local population requirements. Some of these objectives may conflict with both the Clinical Nurse Specialist's objectives and those of other customers, and prioritisation is necessary along with an occasional change in direction. If the local GP fundholders' practice is intent on preventing admissions to hospital for certain interventions and the Clinical Nurse Specialist relied on these admissions as a source of referral, there will be a need to revisit the community element of the role. Although the concept of competition may be an anathema to many specialists, it is well worth the effort to assess the services nurses in other units are providing to determine whether or not a colleague has a competitive edge.

Roof: professional requirements

To concentrate on the first floor would be like leaving the roof off the house, as the chances are that patient expectations and purchaser requirements miss some crucial professional issues. When once asked what standards should be written for nursing practice, it occurred to the author that if nurses just met those defined in statute, there would be plenty to be getting on with. This section cannot linger in this vein for fear of repeating previous chapters, but this much must be said: it is vital that the Clinical Nurse Specialists are clear about their role and its advanced standing. When working at such a senior level the Clinical Nurse Specialist should offer more than an excellent quality of care to a few patients. Within the melting pot of objectives, a reasonable weight should be given to the advancement of the practice of nursing with a necessary emphasis on research and the development of quality tools.

By now the specialist should have a fairly comprehensive mix of objectives and can move on to resource identification.

Bricks: resources

The question is, what resources are required to achieve the objectives? There is a need to identify the roles of other providers in meeting the service objectives from community nurses to acute unit medical staff, and how in all of this the specialist's skills can best be utilised. In other words, where does the Clinical Nurse Specialist fit into the grand plan and which resource mix will achieve the best end result. Quite clearly, the nurse cannot achieve it all alone, although it may sometimes feel that way. Clinical Nurse Specialists are however a small cog in a very big wheel of service provision and their inputs have to be rationed.

From the full complete service across the whole client group, to meeting the needs of just a few, there is a need to put a price on care. Gardner (1992) suggests there are two reasons why the Clinical Nurse Specialist should be 'cost savvy'. First,

> "to influence patient care quality while planning for and responding to cost containment initiatives that interface with nursing practice and second, to influence organisational outcomes by documenting and demonstrating the contribution of the CNS role toward meeting the organisational goal of balancing quality and cost."

At this point it is worth remembering that a service has to have a fairly equal balance of volume, quality and cost, and it may be difficult to sell the concept of a few patients treated at a high price. The Clinical Nurse Specialist should try to define the quality units per patient. Does the service offer one quality unit per patient for 3000 patients or 10 units of quality for just 30 and if the latter, how many other patients go 'unspecialised'? In reality, what would be the cost per patient if only 30 patients per year were specialised and how much can the purchasers be expected to pay for the quality element of a product?

The contention is not to suggest that the Clinical Nurse Specialists spread themselves too thinly as this could incur poor quality, but co-opting others to help achieve the objectives opens the specialist service to more clients and brings down the cost of quality care. Getting the balance between cost, volume and quality (Figure 6.2) is what is required.

The concept of cost containment has been described as incorporating two basic ideas: identifying the best patient outcomes and mobilising and coordinating appropriate resource utilisation (DeZell *et al.*, 1988). A case management approach can be adopted in order to add some structure to the process of care (Nugent, 1992) or alternatively the principle of a value chain can be applied to the patient trail in order that

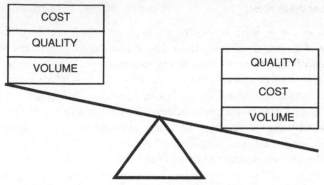

Figure 6.2   *The cost, quality and volume balance*

resource inputs critical to a successful outcome are identified and costed (Johnson and Scholes, 1988).

EVALUATING THE IMPACT: EVALUATING THE OBJECTIVES

> "With no trail for evaluation, accountability is impossible and no budgetary defense exists for maintaining well-paid clinical experts who disappear in a cloud of dust leaving hospital administrators asking, what does a clinical nurse specialist do?"
>
> Malone (1986)

It is, not surprisingly, fairly difficult to measure the effectiveness of the Clinical Nurse Specialist role, but this is exactly what is required. After all, how much implicit goodness can the purchaser be expected to buy (see Figure 6.3)?

The key to evaluation is to find a range of indicators that reflect the scope and objectives of the role. The specialists objectives should now show a span of factors capable of measurement from the most simple

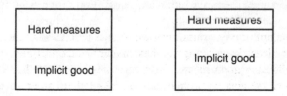

Figure 6.3   *Hard measures and implicit good*

analysis of time between referral and consultation, to the more complex evaluation of outcome.

The more straightforward indicators include:

- Numbers of patients seen and for what;
- Clinics held;
- Domiciliary visits made;
- Referrals and their appropriateness;
- Waiting times to first appointment;
- Cancelled appointments;
- GP communication time delays.

Clearly these are not enough and may not say much about what the Clinical Nurse Specialist perceives to be quality. But this is all about finding a range of indicators that reflect the objectives. Surely every Nurse Specialist sees patients and yet it is surprising how few regularly report on numbers seen and why. This may seem too black and white and it is true to say that not all quality can be measured neatly and reported quarterly, but it is a very important start. However, don't be tempted to stay at measuring the simple indicators: at some stage the Specialist is going to have to move towards outcomes. It may be acceptable initially to report on the number of patients taught self-care techniques, but at some stage the Clinical Nurse Specialist has to ask to what end.

Of course the joy is that having started with the definition of objectives, this process becomes much easier. For instance, if a key objective relates to ensuring appropriate diabetic management at ward level, then measure this by surveying the appropriateness of insulin prescriptions in the wards. If one of the objectives for cardiac rehabilitation concerns the incidence of future infarcts, then trail patients for re-admissions. If an objective gives priority to good stoma management, measure the incidence of skin damage.

Occasionally, process indicators can be used. Ching and Seto (1990) use the process of giving catheter care as an evaluation tool and although this cannot necessarily be linked to outcome, it is certainly a start in the right direction. This example highlights the possibility of using nursing records as a means to evaluation. Although one cannot say that a good care plan means good care, the presence of, say, nutritional assessment in the nursing notes may be a way of assessing the outcome of a staff nurse training programme. A review of the nursing literature offers a number of indicators from re-admissions and length of stay (Russell, 1989; Wade and Moyer, 1989; Ahrens and Padwojski, 1990) to sepsis rates (Field, 1992), and some authors offer guidance as to a complete measurement package (Anderson et al., 1989; Houston and Luquire, 1991) although it should be noted that an off-the-shelf approach may not relate to the Clinical Nurse Specialist's customer objectives.

THE DIFFICULTY OF OUTCOMES

The search for measurable outcomes that determine the quality of the input of any one individual is like the search for the Holy Grail and may end up with as much disappointment. The reality is that it is extremely difficult if not impossible to determine any one individual effect on outcome just as it is difficult to determine the effects of health education on the change in attitude of the recipient. This problem is highlighted by Wade and Moyer (1989) who suggest alternative indicators of patients' knowledge, patient problem solving ability and technical skill, independence, appropriateness of appliances as well as the more standard measurements of length of stay and re-admissions. As stated previously, it will be said that these outcomes are related to many different factors, and it is not appropriate to set up control studies in order to prove a point. However, provided the potential variables at work in the findings are understood, it is quite safe to proceed. Quite clearly many measures are patient orientated and thus will take time to evaluate. A structured programme of feedback is required that does not attempt to evaluate the whole service in one patient encounter. Research skills now come into their own as uninformed patient surveys can be done rather badly. The Clinical Nurse Specialist will require an understanding of the various processes that can be used (Rice *et al.*, 1990).

In the final analysis it will become necessary to move towards the measurement of health gain and the concept of adding life to years or years to life (Evans *et al.*, 1991). It could well be that some of the previous indicators discussed can help along this path, that is, numbers of hospital admissions per individual and measures of independence, and there are health profile tools that can be applied. It perhaps only remains to say that measurement is only as good as the number of people informed of its findings. Consequently there needs to be a sharp increase in the number of Clinical Nurse Specialists writing for publication in order that knowledge can be shared in this vital area of evaluating the impact of nursing.

This chapter has tried to offer a plan of action to help Clinical Nurse Specialists define their service objectives and evaluate their role. The reason that a comprehensive list of off-the-shelf measurement criteria has been excluded is because this points the specialist in the wrong direction. Equally, it may have been noticed that the chapter did not discuss the lengthy process of writing nursing standards. Hopefully this chapter has opened an alternative door: that of the identification of service standards set in conjunction with customers and purchasers, offering a more straightforward and business-like approach to the evaluation of quality.

REFERENCES

Ahrens T.S. and Padwojski A. (1990) Economic effectiveness of an advanced nurse clinician model. *Nursing Management*, 21(11); Critical Care Management Edition): 72J, 72N, 72P.

Anderson E., McCartney E., Schreiber J. and Thompson E. (1989) Productivity measurement for Clinical Nurse Specialists. *Clinical Nurse Specialist*, 3(2): 80–84.

Carter S. and Mowad L. (1988). Is nursing ready for consumerism? *Nursing Administration Quarterly*, 12(3): 74–78.

Ching T.Y. and Seto W.H. (1990) Evaluating the efficacy of the infection control liaison nurse in the hospital. *Journal of Advanced Nursing*, 15(10): 1128–1131.

Department of Health (1991a) *The Health of the Nation: A Strategy for Health in England, Cm1523*. HMSO, London.

Department of Health (1991b) *The Patients' Charter: Raising the Standard*. HMSO, London.

DeZell A., Comeau E. and Zander K. (1988) *Patients and Purse Strings: Nursing Case Management: Managed Care via the Nursing Care Management Model*. National League for Nursing, NLN Publications 20–2191, Vol. 2, pp. 253–264.

Eriksen L. (1987). Patient satisfaction: an indicator of nursing care quality? *Nursing Management* 18(7): 31–35.

Evans D., Evans M. and Greaves D. (1991). Adding life to years: problems in planning for health gain. *International Journal of Health Care Quality Assurance*, 4(1): 13–20.

Field J. (1992) A specialist role in patient nutrition. *Nursing Standard*, 6(38): 38–39.

Gardner D. (1992) The CNS as a cost manager. *Clinical Nurse Specialist*, 6(2): 112–115.

Houston S. and Luquire R. (1991) Measuring success: CNS performance appraisal. *Clinical Nurse Specialist*, 5(4): 204–209.

Johnson G. and Scholes K. (1988) *Exploring Corporate Strategy*, 2nd edn. Prentice-Hall, Englewood Cliffs, New Jersey.

Kakabadse A., Ludlow R. and Vinnicombe S. (1988) *Working in Organisations*. Penguin Business, Harmondsworth, Middlesex.

Malone B.L. (1986) Working with people: evaluation of the Clinical Nurse Specialist. *American Journal of Nursing*, 86(12): 1375–1377.

Nugent K. (1992) The clinical nurse specialist as case manager in a collaborative practice model: bridging the gap between quality and cost of care. *Clinical Nurse Specialist*, 6(2): 106–111.

Rice J., Wegmiller D. and Laslow L. (1990) Patient satisfaction monitoring within a comprehensive quality management system. *International Journal of Health Care Quality Assurance*, 3(4): 18–26.

Russell L. (1989) Cost containment of modified radical mastectomy: the impact of the clinical nurse specialist. *Point of View*, 26(3): 18–19.

Shatzman L. and Strauss A.L. (1973) *Field Research*. Prentice-Hall, Englewood Cliffs, New Jersey.

Smith M. (1990) Making the most of the CNS. *Senior Nurse*, 10(9): 6–8.

Wade B. and Moyer A. (1989) An evaluation of clinical nurse specialists: implications for education and the organisation of care. *Senior Nurse*, 9(9): 11–16.

Wilson C. (1988) The impact of utilisation review programs on consumer expectations, decision making, and access to health care. *Nursing Administration Quarterly*, 12(3): 51–56.

CHAPTER SEVEN

The nurse consultant: fact or fiction?

Stephen Graham Wright

INTRODUCTION – A BACKGROUND OF UNCERTAINTY

A growing body of nurses in the United Kingdom (UK) has now adopted the title 'Consultant Nurse' or 'Nurse Consultant'. These two terms are themselves symptomatic of a wider lack of clarity about what constitutes the role. Some nurses appear to have roles that are Consultant Nurses (and for the sake of simplicity, this is the preferred term which will be used in this chapter) yet whose titles do not suggest this directly (for example, Senior Nurse – Clinical Practice Development). There appears to be no clear consensus as to what constitutes the role of Consultant Nurses, what their functions are, what educational background or experience they should have, what pay scales are appropriate, or how they differ from other, but clearly related, roles such as the Clinical Nurse Specialist.

As yet, no research specifying the role of the Consultant Nurse has emerged in the UK; and the title seems to have been applied to a wide range of nursing occupations. A scan through the job advertisement section of journals may suggest Consultant Nurse roles with emphases in marketing (for manufacturers of drugs and medical equipment), research assistant (medical research programmes) or in giving professional advice to health-orientated bodies and authorities. In addition, a considerable number of nurses have set up independent enterprises, partnerships or companies where nurse consultants offer nurse consultancy – usually in the fields of management, educational and organisational development. Meanwhile, Pearson (1983), Wright (1986) and Wright *et al.* (1991) have identified Consultant Nurse roles which are dominated by the emphasis on clinical practice input.

Furthermore, the act of consultancy does not appear to be exclusive to one role. For example, consultancy in the form of giving specialist advice may form part of the everyday work of a nurse manager, community nurse, nurse specialist, nurse teacher and ward sister/charge nurse. The Consultant Nurse, therefore, cannot lay sole claim to the act of consultancy in nursing. Indeed, the roles of the Consultant Nurse and its close relative the Clinical Nurse Specialist are often difficult to distinguish – perhaps not least because as the nurse specialist role evolves, it has developed more and more into one of consultancy. However, while others may have an element of consultancy in their jobs, for the Consultant Nurse it is the dominant activity, the *raison d'être*.

At first sight, this lack of consensus and definition may seem somewhat messy and uncertain, leaving the role open to misinterpretation and unfair exploitation. At the same time, a lack of defining the boundaries also prevents them from being confined. Thus there is enormous potential to develop roles in many flexible ways, which can be of considerable benefit both to patients/clients and the wider organisation. In this sense, the Consultant Nurse role appears to be following that of many others, as predicted by Toffler (1973). With less emphasis on permanency of post and job description, there is a growing trend to the creation of *ad hoc* flexible roles, able to respond to a variety of situations and needs.

THE NATURE OF CONSULTANCY AND THE CONSULTANT NURSE ROLE

Allen (1990) offers some help in defining the consultant and the nature of consultancy. A consultant is "a person providing professional advice etc., especially for a fee." Difficulties might then arise in defining who or what is 'professional.' Indeed the word 'consultant' like 'professional' is now used widely in many fields so that attempts at strict definition of terms can become meaningless. For example, the dictionary goes on to refer to a consultant as "a senior specialist in a branch of medicine responsible for patients in hospital."

However the concept of the 'consultant' has now been taken up widely in relation to many occupations, for example consultant engineer, marketing consultant and management consultant. Anecdotal evidence for some early UK consultant nurses (Wright *et al.*, 1991) suggests that some senior medical staff have reacted negatively to the use of the term 'consultants' with nurses. However, this would not appear to have been a significantly widespread phenomenon. The generally accepted use of the word in many areas of employment has further eroded any remaining claims to exclusive use of the title.

Two elements seem to be significant which are worthy of discussion at this stage. Firstly, is the consultant being used to imply status above other groups? Secondly, does the term adequately convey a particular nurses function? It may simply be that, in using the word to describe a particular function, it helps some nurses in busy organisations to identify what someone does. Others who see the title as reinforcing hierarchical authority, such as some medical specialists, might indeed be sensitive when others adopt the word into their own occupations. How far nurses, who have a long history of hierarchical titles and chains of command, will use the word 'consultant' to convey status, superiority and power over others has yet to be seen. Hopefully, this will not be the case, and is unlikely to become so if the way the consultant operates develops in the ways advocated later in this chapter, essentially one of working in a partnership relationship, not master–servant, with patients and nurses.

Some other questions need to be asked about this 'giving professional advice' by the consultant. How far is the consultant involved with the person seeking advice and the setting or issue to which it is applied? On what knowledge basis does the consultant give advice, do we accept that the consultant possesses a certain specialist body of knowledge, and if so, how can this be proven and demonstrated? To give advice suggests that a certain 'take it or leave it' quality exists. Thus the consultant may have little or no executive authority to ensure that a suggestion is carried through. On the other hand, the consultants, because of their perceived greater body of knowledge, experience and wisdom carry considerable sapiential authority, that is 'I can't *tell* you what to do, because I'm not your manager, but if you ignore my advice, which you sought, and which is based on my experience and breadth and depth of knowledge, then there may be serious consequences for you and/or your patient'.

Thus, the nature of the advice being sought, the level of expertise of the consultant and the involvement of the consultants in the issue on which advice is being sought, are three interacting factors which will affect profoundly the way in which the consultant works. In examining the *modus operandi* of different types of consultant nurse, it seems that four principal approaches are in use in nursing, as discussed below.

Nurse-centred consultations

Here a ward sister or charge nurse, or a nurse working in the patient's home, for example, may seek advice about the specific management of a patient's problem. Advice is given to the nurse, who may then incorporate it in the overall management of the patient's care. The consultant here is involved primarily with the nurse and may have little, if any, contact with the patient. For example, a nurse on an acute surgical ward may telephone a consultant nurse in a Care of the Elderly Unit for advice. An elderly patient may be presenting specific problems about which the surgical nurse is uncertain, the advice may take place only over the telephone, and there is no obligation on the part of the surgical nurse to follow it. Referring also to the dictionary definitions mentioned earlier, it may also be questioned whether a 'fee' has been paid. In the above example, it would be unlikely that the surgical nurse paid a fee! However, the employing authority would presumably pay the consultant's salary, with an understanding that the role was used to advise a wide variety of staff.

Patient-centred forms

In some settings, advice to nurses may also encompass working directly with patients: a consultancy such as this draws on the consultant's expertise and involves them in patient care, perhaps acting as a role model, demonstrating a specialist technique or helping with the care plan.

Education-centred

Many Consultant Nurses are involved in developing courses, conferences and workshops for staff, and such education-centred forms of consultancy are becoming increasingly common. The consultant may actively participate in carrying through the teaching/development of the programme.

Management-centred

This form of consultancy is also fairly common, here the Consultant Nurse gives advice on organisational development, role identification, nursing policies and so on.

While organisations may employ staff in specific consultant roles to carry out the above work, it seems to be increasingly common for nurses to work as independent consultants, and charge fees for their advice. Clearly, consultations in management and education lend themselves far more easily to independent consultation, rather than, say, those forms affecting nursing practice which are more likely to be spontaneous and short-lived requests for advice. It is also evident that acting as a consultant is not exclusive to the Consultant Nurse role. Many others, such as Clinical Nurse Specialists, would lay claim to this territory and might find a role for themselves in all the examples given above. However, both Clinical Nurse Specialists and Consultant Nurses have a variety of functions, but it is the role of the latter for whom consultation is the principle activity – indeed its *raison d'être*.

THE KNOWLEDGE AND SKILL BASE FOR THE CONSULTANT NURSE

Many nurses can be involved in acts of consultation, but several features mark out the Consultant Nurse role as somewhat different. Firstly, the principle occupational activity is one of consultancy – it may not be exclusively so, but it dominates a large part of the Consultant Nurse's working life. Secondly, working almost exclusively in a consultancy capacity implies that a particular level of knowledge and expertise has been achieved. While this knowledge and expertise may have its basis in a particular speciality, the Consultant Nurse has a greater breadth of understanding of nursing issues in general. The Clinical Nurse Specialist, for example, may focus on a particular client group with specialist problems, for example a Diabetes Nurse Specialist. The Consultant Nurse has an expanded knowledge base and skill at work in the wide territory of nursing – its political, social and organisational context, its broad theoretical base, and so on. Thus the Consultant Nurse may not only be linked to a particular speciality, but may offer across the board advice on a wide range of nursing issues in an organisation, and may offer advice, perhaps for a fee, to external organisations.

Caplan (1970) and Menard (1987) see the Consultant Nurse as an expert teacher, able to facilitate a wide range of educational programmes, from one-to-one teaching, to group work, conference work, curriculum and programme development. Wright (1986) and Pearson (1983) have argued strongly that the consultant should have extensive expertise and knowledge in a particular speciality, that they should still have a hands-on role in nursing practice to enhance clinical credibility and the ability to work as an effective role model. The Consultant Nurse is also a confident autonomous practitioner and able to be such because of the breadth and depth of knowledge actually possessed. They all see the consultant as having a significant and explicit role as a change agent, facilitating staff development and creativity, questioning and evaluating practice and challenging established norms. Consultant Nurses are expert communicators able to get information across both verbally and in writing. As such they possess an entrepreneurial ability to develop their role and market their skills to the advantage of the organisation and the development of nursing practice.

Benner (1984) sees the consultant as having achieved the level of 'expert' nurse and educator to at least Masters Degree level. Clearly this has implications for the support and development of all nurses if sufficient numbers of this calibre are to emerge. Such nurses are 'connoisseurs' of nursing and the system in which they work. The consultant is an expert in understanding how the organisation 'ticks' and how to use a variety of creative ways of getting around the bureaucracy to meet the needs of patients and their carers, and the goals of nursing. Benner (1984) also suggests that the role is "unclear and more complex" than can be defined by a job description, as the expert nurse links both formally and informally to affect practice, and is involved in both monitoring and evaluating care. Thus, to support this wide range of interventions and activities, the Consultant Nurse needs a considerable body of knowledge and skill, backed up with a broad range of interpersonal, managerial and research skills. The Consultant Nurse is able to act as a leader in his or her field, helping to set a vision for nursing and motivate nurses towards it; and to facilitate the process of change as it becomes necessary.

There are other qualities which Consultant Nurses must possess to fulfil their function. This is more than the possession of experience or certificates, indeed some might argue they are their foundations. Without them, the experience and the paper qualifications may be evidence of mere time-serving or pen-pushing! From the literature cited earlier, a number of features can be defined to help build up a kind of picture of what sort of person the Consultant Nurse is. Underpinning their experience and qualifications must be:

- good communication verbally/in writing;
- mature judgement/problem solving skills;
- physical and psychological stamina;
- political awareness getting around the bureaucracy;
- analytical thinking abilities;
- ability to use intuition and initiative;
- awareness of self (abilities, limitations);
- high level of commitment to nurses and to nursing.

To assist with these the Consultant Nurse needs: social, domestic and peer group support, practice role models of their own, and adequate administration and secretarial support to do the work.

Thus, high demands and expectations are made of the Consultant Nurse role and the person who occupies it. The principal modes have been described: the detached advisor, offering help with the 'take it or leave it' quality attached and the involved clinician. It is this latter approach which is espoused by Pearson (1983) and Wright (1986) as the most significant in effecting changes in nursing practice and in reducing the risks of Consultant Nurse roles emerging on an elite group, standing aside, uncontaminated by the messy world of direct care.

The consultant, in being clinically involved, is a move away from the model of the consultant as an aloof and uncommitted figure. Encouraging learning, motivating nurses, sharing expertise and acting as a role model for others can only take place in a setting which positively encourages these behaviours. Being directly involved in the work place and working as a 'hands on' nurse with colleagues enables the consultant to retain clinical credibility and to be instrumental in producing an appropriate climate for learning and innovation and the achievement of high quality care. All of this is essential if nurses are to meet the requirements of the Post Registration Education Project (United Kingdom Central Council, 1990) and be encouraged to see learning as a way of life.

The ability to demonstrate excellence in practice and the opportunity to bring to the clinical setting the expertise that can only be acquired over many years of learning are fundamental to the value and role of the Consultant Nurse. To be divorced from practice would expose the consultant to the risk of being seen as an 'ivory tower' nurse, reinforcing, not bridging, the gap between the theory and practice of nursing. Where the Consultant Nurse has a role which aspires to having immediate effects upon practice, and those nurses involved in it, then it is essential that they remain a clinician. This might take the form of working with nurses and patients over quite long periods of time and perhaps taking full responsibility for the care of some patients as a primary or associate nurse. Whatever the method chosen, having some degree of accountability for patient care puts the Consultant Nurse in the best position to influence practice.

Producing a climate for learning, innovation and patient-centred practice is, therefore, central to the Consultant Nurse's role. When such a climate is not achieved the ramifications go beyond the effects upon staff learning. The Price Waterhouse report (1988) mirrors that of the American 'Magnet' study (McClure et al., (1983) in suggesting that a climate which is hostile to learning, which does not support innovative, patient-centred practice, and where managers and other leaders do not actively support the staff ultimately fails both nurses and patients. Care tends to decline to an institutional mould, and staff demonstrate their dissatisfaction with poor motivation and high sickness, absenteeism and leaving rates. Potential recruits can easily sense such a negative climate, and will seek work elsewhere; highly motivated individuals who already work there will tend not to stay long. Nursing has a great need for 'clinical leaders' to produce environments for creativity on a mass scale (Rafferty, 1993) in all areas of nursing. Both nurses and nursing, and ultimately patients, would benefit by exposure to more nurses who can demonstrate expertise and excellence in their fields.

NURSING ENTREPRENEURS

The creative, adaptable practitioner, that is the Consultant Nurse, is able to transcend the boundaries of any job description. Indeed, it may be argued that the ability to use a job description as a launching pad for other initiatives is itself characteristic of the successful consultant nurse.

Clinical grading scales currently are limited in their grades, so it may well be that consultants also have the ability not only to negotiate their way around nursing, but also an appropriate remuneration for their role. Increasingly, in the light of recent health care reforms, more and more nurses are finding that rates of pay are open to negotiation. Clearly, in the hands of unscrupulous employers or where a nurse is not skilled in assertiveness and negotiation, this is a system open to abuse and exploitation. Consultant Nurses have to be very clear about what is needed to secure the best pay and conditions for themselves as a just reward for their work, and to ensure their own continued professional development is achieved.

Consultant Nurses also need to be able to adapt to changes in the health care system, to survive and prosper, if the goals of nursing are to be achieved. Recent trends emphasising the use of market and commercial techniques in health care may put patients and nurses at risk. Consultant Nurses can be in the vanguard of those who are able to argue for the value of nursing, to secure nursing resources and development, and to practise patient-centred forms of care. Organisations which seek to promote patient-centred high quality care, driven by the demands of users of the services and initiatives such as *The Patients' Charter* (Department of Health, 1991), also have to promote themselves in the growing competitiveness of the health care system. Consultant Nurses, with all the skills they possess, may find themselves in increasing demand for advice in service and educational development; and in using their abilities in income generation schemes. Thus they have an important role to play in ensuring that increasing competition in health care is not achieved at the cost of high quality care. The Consultant Nurse can be both ambassador and entrepreneur for nursing, ensuring that quality and caring count for as much as quantity and cost-effectiveness.

As nursing developments take place overseas, many UK nurses are finding that they are held in high regard and demand for action and assistance especially in the restructuring countries of Eastern Europe. Independent Consultant Nurses, and nurses employed with the National Health Service, are going up many avenues of much needed nursing development. There is much that can be contributed in the wider international field. For some, especially those in the National Health Service, the work has been seen as an accepted part of their existing role, and supported by employers who wish to develop links with other European countries. Others may explore appropriate avenues which may generate income for the employer while others may strike out along a totally independent path. Both inside and outside the National Health Service, and inside and outside the UK, there is no doubt that there is a growing demand for health-care professionals who have developed effective entrepreneurial skills – entrepreneurial skills to benefit themselves, their employing organisations and nursing. Such a survivor in the system can be a real force for change, as well as someone well placed to ensure that the value of high-quality patient-centred care receives a high profile and success.

CONCLUSION

The Consultant Nurse role, if properly developed and supported, seems to be in an ideal position to extend the boundaries of nursing, to act as a role model for excellence in practice, to provide high quality patient care and higher morale among staff, with its consequence for matters of recruitment and retention. The consultants have a clear vision and 'image' in their heads of what nursing is, which they can draw upon to effect expert practice to the benefit of both their clients and colleagues.

The role as outlined, is more than a means of a lift up the grading ladder or the performance of complex technical skills. The role, among a number of others such as clinical specialists, primary nurse or lecturer practitioner, is in the vanguard of those nurses who are testing out the boundaries of the territory of nursing. They are expanding their knowledge and skill into a wide range of health care activities and demonstrating the importance and value of nursing in all of them.

The Consultant Nurse role is not a panacea for nursing's ills, but it is a growing reality for more and more nurses. Its arrival has been evolutionary rather than revolutionary and its activities need far more research and a clearer definition. In the meantime, it remains a role of enormous range and potential which many nurses can find challenging and rewarding. Through it, they can make a real contribution to improving the quality of patient care, ensuring that the role is fact not fiction.

REFERENCES

Allen R.E. (Ed.) (1990) *The Concise Oxford English Dictionary.* Clarendon, Oxford.

Benner P. (1984) *From Novice to Expert.* Addison-Wesley, Menlo Park, California.

Caplan G. (1970) *The Theory and Practice of Mental Health Consultation.* Basic Books, New York.

Department of Health (1991) *The Patients' Charter: Raising the Standard.* HMSO, London.

McClure M.L., Poulin M.A., Sovie M.D. and Wandelt M.A. (1983) *Magnet Hospitals – Attraction and Retention of Professional Nurses.* American Academy of Nursing, Kansas City.

Menard S.W. (1987) *The Clinical Nurse Specialist – Perspective on Practice.* Wiley, New York.

Pearson A. (1983) *The Clinical Nursing Unit.* Heinemann, London.

Price Waterhouse (1988) *Nurse Retention and Recruitment.* Price Waterhouse, London.

Rafferty A-M. (1993) *Leading Questions.* King's Fund Institute, London.

Toffler A. (1973) *Future Shock.* Pan, London.

United Kingdom Central Council (1990) *Post Registration Education Project.* UKCC, London.

Wright S.G. (1986) *Building and Using a Model at Nursing.* Arnold, London.

Wright S.G., Johnson M.L.J. and Purdy E. (1991) The nurse as a consultant. *Nursing Standard,* 5(20): 31–34.